This book is a valuable resource for therapists working in communities and with communities to address a variety of urgent psychosocial challenges, such as improving race relations, reducing political polarization, and promoting peer support in health care. At a time when citizen participation is so needed to strengthen our democracy, therapists will find this book helpful as a guide to expanding their role to include education, advocacy, and organizing for community-based problem solving.

—**Jack Saul, PhD**, author of *Collective Trauma, Collective Healing: Promoting Community Resilience in the Aftermath of Disaster*

Doherty and Mendenhall bring therapy and democracy together in an inspiring handbook that encourages all of us to become "citizen therapists." They vividly describe real-life partnerships and collaborations between therapists and community members in which *each person* has expertise and energy to bring to community problems. The chapters include collective efforts focused on serious problems of our time, such as chronic illness, political polarization, and relations between police and young Black men. Are you feeling helpless in our current fragmented world? Has the COVID experience and political polarization rendered you pessimistic and passive? I strongly encourage you to *read this book*! Doherty and Mendenhall's concept of "citizen therapist" is an inspiring recipe for reengaging our collective sense of agency, communion, and hope.

—**Susan H. McDaniel, PhD**, Dr. Laurie Sands Distinguished Professor of Families & Health, Academic Chief, Division of Collaborative Care and Wellness, and Director of the Institute for the Family in the Department of Psychiatry, University of Rochester, Rochester, NY

BECOMING A CITIZEN THERAPIST

BECOMING A CITIZEN THERAPIST

Integrating Community
Problem-Solving
Into Your Work
as a Healer

WILLIAM J. DOHERTY | TAJ J. MENDENHALL

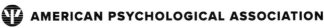 AMERICAN PSYCHOLOGICAL ASSOCIATION

Published by
American Psychological Association
750 First Street, NE
Washington, DC 20002
https://www.apa.org

Order Department
https://www.apa.org/pubs/books
order@apa.org

Typeset in Charter and Interstate by Circle Graphics, Inc., Reisterstown, MD

Printer: Gasch Printing, Odenton, MD
Cover Designer: Anne Kerns, Anne Likes Red, Inc., Silver Spring, MD

Library of Congress Cataloging-in-Publication Data

Names: Doherty, William J. (William Joseph), 1945- author. |
    Mendenhall, Tai, author.
Title: Becoming a citizen therapist : integrating community problem-solving
    into your work as a healer / William J. Doherty and Tai J. Mendenhall.
Description: Washington, DC : American Psychological Association, [2024] |
    Includes bibliographical references and index.
Identifiers: LCCN 2023027455 (print) | LCCN 2023027456 (ebook) |
    ISBN 9781433839863 (paperback) | ISBN 9781433839870 (ebook)
Subjects: LCSH: Community psychology. | Community mental health services. |
    Psychotherapy--Social aspects.
Classification: LCC RA790.55 .D64 2024 (print) | LCC RA790.55 (ebook) |
    DDC 362.2/2--dc23/eng/20230912
LC record available at https://lccn.loc.gov/2023027455
LC ebook record available at https://lccn.loc.gov/2023027456

https://doi.org/10.1037/0000378-000

Printed in the United States of America

10 9 8 7 6 5 4 3 2 1

Contents

PART I OVERVIEW OF CITIZEN THERAPIST WORK

INTRODUCTION

What Can Therapists Offer the Larger World?

As someone who came of age in the 1960s, I (Bill) viewed therapists as potential change agents in society. If we got enough political leaders into personal growth groups, would social justice not be far away? Fast forward to the mid-1990s when I had become deeply dissatisfied with the constricted role of therapists in an increasingly troubled world. I was haunted by Hillman and Ventura's (1993) classic book, *We've Had a Hundred Years of Psychotherapy—and the World's Getting Worse.* Looking back, I realized that my training in the humanistic psychology era of the 1970s had left me with the naïve notion that widespread uptake of therapy and related self-help offerings would bubble up to change the larger society. Likewise, my deep dive into family systems theory had left me with unrealistic expectations of how family therapy principles could apply to the broader systems of society.

My training took place in a long-gone era of optimism when the world seemed to be newly discovering psychology and the fruits of therapy. But by the end of the 1970s, the Equal Rights Amendment had stalled, the divorce rate had doubled, violent crime was escalating, indicators of social trust had begun their decline, and the economy was mired in something called *stagflation* (Bailey & Farber, 2004). The Reagan era of the 1980s would dash

https://doi.org/10.1037/0000378-001
Becoming a Citizen Therapist: Integrating Community Problem-Solving Into Your Work as a Healer, by W. J. Doherty and T. J. Mendenhall

hopes that national leaders would welcome the application of therapy and the social sciences for solving our social problems.

As I looked around for models of how to work as a therapist on social change and community well-being, I was not comforted. The prevailing community psychology models seemed to disparage therapy practitioners as offering Band-Aids for problems that were structural, not personal (Albee, 1998). The real answers, we therapists were told, would come from public policy experts, legislative advocates, and community specialists with expertise in public, large-scale projects. Meaningful action was upstream—to prevent mental health problems—and therapists worked downstream via the medical model of treating people after they developed diagnosable problems.

Would I have to abandon my clinical work and identity as a therapist if I wanted to make a difference in the broader community? It seemed too late in my career for that kind of transition; I was an experienced, enthusiastic therapist and midcareer academic. The community-change projects I knew about involved large grants or public funds to hire community psychologists or community social workers, with no role for therapists. Our contributions were relegated to offering pro bono services or practicing in economically disadvantaged communities. Or maybe write a book for the lay public. (Nowadays, it would be to write a popular blog or have a social media account with lots of followers.)

Then, as now, the most accessible way to become involved in the public sphere was via advocacy for the profession: protecting licensure, gaining access to the insurance panels, and obtaining favorable reimbursement rates. All legitimate endeavors but not exactly world changing. Success in the policy arena generally depends on raising funds and hiring good lobbyists. Although important for the profession, this kind of advocacy comes with an unspoken assumption that if therapists thrive in the clinical practice of psychotherapy, the world will do better. We now have more than 100 years of data that only partially support this assumption. We do help many people, but we don't seem to be counteracting a toxic environment, let alone forging new pathways for people to connect to their communities and solve social problems.

BREAKING THROUGH TO A WIDER VIEW

Staying with Bill's story for now (Tai's story comes later): By the mid-1990s, I had finished writing a book on the ethical and moral dimensions of psychotherapy (Doherty, 1995), in which I challenged the field to move beyond a nearly exclusive emphasis on the individual self-interest of the client. (Doherty, 2022, is an updated version of that book.) I called for considering additional stakeholders in clients' actions and decisions, including family members and others closely connected to the client. The book included a chapter on community because I did not want to limit the ethical dimension of life to personal relationships. But my ideas there were underdeveloped. I had defined the aspiration that therapists might promote community well-being, but I did not yet have a guiding map.

That map came from outside of our field via mentoring by political theorists and social activists Harry Boyte and Nancy Kari, who were connected to the University of Minnesota's Center for Democracy and Citizenship. (See Chapter 1 of this book for an explanation of their public work model.) As I turned the pages of the typed, prepublication version of their new book (Boyte & Kari, 1996), I told myself, "This is where I want to take my career now." They gave me a critique of traditional professionalism as it emerged in the early 20th century and a way of thinking about how a professional can be an agent of community capacity building and grassroots democracy. I felt the same kind of thrill as when I first engaged with the world of psychology and family therapy.

This thrill came with discomfort because it meant a reevaluation of my identity as a therapist and academic. I realized that I had always seen my work as apart from community, even above it, as something delivered to community and not done alongside community. My fellow citizens were the population I served, taught, and studied, not my partners in solving problems. As a therapist I helped clients access their personal capacities, but I never considered how I might help groups of citizens access their collective capacities for promoting mutual well-being and solving public problems. (Note: In this book we use the term *citizens* not in its legal sense but to refer to joint stakeholders in building and maintaining communities and the larger commonwealth.)

But where to start? Along with colleague Patrick Dougherty, I launched a local group of therapists to explore the possibilities of deeper engagement with our community. Although launched with a big goal and the lofty name "The Psychotherapy and Public Work Project," it was a bust. We couldn't agree on what kind of project to work on, and nobody but Patrick and I was interested in reading Boyte and Kari's book. In retrospect, the most problematic part was that we seemed to think of public engagement as engaging with low-income, ethnic minority communities. And we were all White professionals in either private practice or big institutions such as hospitals or universities, with little access to the communities we assumed we should be working with. After that group dissolved, I realized that I would have to set out on my own to learn to be what I would later come to call a "citizen therapist" and to start with communities I did have access to.

Because I had a background in codeveloping the area of medical family therapy (McDaniel et al., 2014), I decided to start my citizen therapist journey around a health care problem that was taxing the care system and the communities it served. Through the influence of physician colleague Mac Baird, I approached the health promotion leaders of HealthPartners, a large health care organization. The idea was to engage patients as leaders to codevelop a project that would draw on their capacities to make a difference for fellow patients. Furthermore, I offered to work pro bono on the project. The HealthPartners leaders were intrigued. I asked them what problem they would like to start with, and they chose diabetes for a variety of reasons (chronic, difficult to manage, many complications, and expensive to the health care system). They put out the word to the clinics they thought might be interested, and a clinic leader, physician Jim Hart, stepped up.

Around this time, I met my coauthor, Tai, a graduate student who was exploring medical family therapy as a potential career specialty. Within a couple of months, Tai and I were meeting with a group of clinic patients who were experienced with diabetes and eager to share their expertise. The year was 1999, and this was my internship with citizen therapist work. More than 2 decades later, I haven't stopped engaging with fellow citizens across a variety of other settings to cocreate and carry out the projects described in this book. Next Tai will tell his origin story in this work.

TAI'S STORY

I was in graduate school when I began to be disillusioned with traditional models in academia and therapy. I had finished my master of science degree in marriage and family therapy, during which time I had fallen in love with systems theory. My dissatisfaction stemmed from three observations about the models I was learning to practice. First, the therapist was positioned as the unquestioned expert, delivering care in a top-down, provider–consumer manner and functioning in isolation from other professions. Second, clients were portrayed as having straightforward mental health or relational troubles, and medical and larger community issues were rarely mentioned or attended to. Third, we never connected clients with one another for mutual learning and support; instead, they waited their turn to get treated by a professional. As much as I loved seeing clients, therapy as a profession seemed too hierarchical and too limited in scope.

In 1999, I began my doctoral studies and declared medical family therapy as a specialization in my journey. I sought out Bill, one of the founders of this specialization, as my advisor. He helped me get an early clinical placement in a primary care residency, which sealed the deal for me that choosing this path was a good idea. Far from the isolated, structured, 1-hour-at-a-time models of private practice with a relatively narrow range of clients and clinical presentations I had started with in my graduate training, this work was interdisciplinary, collaborative, often unpredictable, diverse, and clinically intense. I engaged with teams that included physicians, mental health providers, social service experts, patient advocates, interpreters, and cultural brokers such as community Elders and shamans.

I recall during the early days of my doctoral program feeling as if I had "arrived." I had finally figured out what I was going to do. My plan: to never leave this messy world of on-the-ground, in-the-trenches, systemic, integrated health care and to continue to advance its mission and scope as a clinician, teacher, trainer, supervisor, and scholar.

But something started to nag at me as I worked harder and harder, especially in cases that involved those who were living with chronic illnesses. I wished that, while offering care, I could consult with some patients and their families who'd dealt with similar issues, to find out what worked best for them. I found myself bumping up against conventional practice patterns where care had to go one way—from me to patients in a provider–consumer direction. But I did not usually have the lived experience and wisdom that other patients had, a wisdom gained by actually having an illness or living with someone with that illness. Instead of sitting in the waiting room looking at outdated magazines or their cellphones, wouldn't it be great if a "veteran patient" could talk with a newly diagnosed one? Or if a spouse who had figured out how to be supportive without being a nag about diet, exercise, and medications could talk with somebody who wanted to be helpful but was not sure how?

I didn't know it then, but Bill was struggling with some of these same challenges related to scope and reach, tapping both professional knowledge and lived-experience knowledge. As mentioned above, he was talking with HealthPartners leaders about ways to engage patients living with diabetes as coleaders to codevelop a project that would draw on their capacities to make a difference for fellow patients, and he invited me into the emerging project. What followed was our first citizen therapist initiative. Its evolution and key learnings were the principal focus of my doctoral dissertation, and it set into motion the career that I have pursued in integrated health care and citizen therapist work ever since.

THE PARTNERS IN DIABETES PROJECT: TAI'S STORY CONTINUES

Bill and I have told the long-version story of our first project—Partners in Diabetes—through a couple of publications (Mendenhall & Doherty, 2003, 2007b). The short version is this: Our early meetings with physicians, clinic administrators, and providers and then with patients and their families served to confirm that diabetes was a pressure point for everybody. Put simply, this meant that nobody was happy with how things were going. Although their reasons were different (administrators were worried about how much diabetes care was costing; providers were wrestling with feelings of futility and being "maxed out"; patients felt demoralized by characterizations of them as noncompliant vis-à-vis commonplace inabilities to afford healthy foods, not feeling safe to exercise in their neighborhoods), everybody agreed that something new was needed.

Providers nominated and invited 14 patients and spouses of patients to coconstruct a project in which they would be paired as support partners with other patients and families who were struggling with diabetes. These paired patients and family members were generally in one of two situations: (a) they were struggling with managing the disease well (e.g., three consecutive A1C tests of > 9%) or (b) they had recently been diagnosed and were thereby navigating initial and often overwhelming phases of adjusting to it. The support partners' efforts involved a variety of diabetes management strategies and educational content. In some cases they met with members once for an encouraging pep talk, and in other cases they met for several months in person or over the telephone.

As a supplement to standard care, patients' engagement with Partners in Diabetes was not billed, and the content of meetings between support partners and members was not formally documented in medical records or related charting. And though the project was not formally evaluated, anecdotally patients and providers communicated high satisfaction with the program. Patients described learning strategies for effective disease management (e.g., administering insulin injections, where and when to purchase healthy foods affordably, chair aerobics at home). Providers described patients whom they had long since given up on to manage diabetes well to be improving across metabolic control, weight, and blood pressure measures. Alongside this, administrators described feeling more hopeful about diabetes not bankrupting their clinic.

For my dissertation, I conducted a thematic analysis of process notes and in-depth, key-informant interviews (Mendenhall & Doherty, 2003, 2007b). In retrospect, this was somewhat risky because the project's planning took many turns and nearly did not come to fruition. The risk was made vividly clear to me when, about halfway through, Bill asked the leadership group of patients and providers if we "still have a project here," given that energy and meeting attendance seemed to be flagging. (The group rose to the challenge and recommitted to the work.) I'm still a bit traumatized by that—this was to be my dissertation!—and have forever since recommended that my own graduate students not do dissertations on startup projects.

In Partners in Diabetes, Bill and I learned how to work with leadership groups that included patients, family members, and providers in a flattened hierarchy. The patients developed confidence in their own wisdom as "life experts." The providers learned a new form of collaboration in which their knowledge and expertise were "on tap," not "on top." Once this democratic process was in place, every decision was made collaboratively: designing support partners' training curriculum, marketing the program, coordinating referral processes, and performing ongoing program troubleshooting and problem solving. And it never took more than 2 to 4 hours per week of anybody's time.

After several years of local implementation across two clinics, Partners in Diabetes concluded when one clinic closed and the other changed its clinical focus. But the project's DNA had already begun to inform other like-minded projects. One, called the ANGELS (A Neighbor Giving Encouragement, Love, and Support), was taking root through my internship placement in a partnership between providers in a children's hospital, adolescent patients, and their parents in North Carolina (Mendenhall & Doherty, 2007a). Another, called the FEDS (Family Education Diabetes Series), was gaining momentum in Saint Paul, Minnesota, through a partnership between an American Indian[1] community organization and the University of Minnesota (Mendenhall et al., 2010). This project, originally proposed by two local Elders who were also support partners in Partners in Diabetes, would go on to be the longest-standing citizen health care project to date (see Chapter 2).

ANOTHER STARTUP PROJECT: PUTTING FAMILY FIRST

Back to Bill now. A second project belongs in the origin story of our citizen therapist work because it began at the same time as Partners in Diabetes and because its very different focus illustrates the breadth of issues that can be tackled through this way of working.

---

[1] We use the terms *American Indian*, *Indigenous*, and *Native* interchangeably. This is consistent with preferences of Elders in the FEDS.

In April 1998, I gave a keynote talk to a large conference for parents in Wayzata, Minnesota—an upper-middle-class suburb of Minneapolis—on the topic of family time and family rituals. I addressed a concern I had been hearing about the loss of family time to outside activities for children and the rat race that parents were experiencing in keeping up with sports practices and traveling teams. The parents responded to the message but were befuddled about how they could buck the trend of overbusyness, given the pressures they felt to have their children succeed. Several school leaders who attended told me privately that their schools were contributing to the problem by offering an ever-increasing array of activities without alerting parents to the side effect: the loss of family time and downtime for kids. The upshot for me was a deeper awareness of the connection between the personal and public dimensions of disappearing family time.

Later that year, the conference organizer invited me to give a similar talk during a new lecture series on parenting. I saw an opportunity to try out my wings as a publicly engaged therapist. I declined to just give a presentation on the same topic but proposed that we organize parents to take action on the problem. She readily agreed. So, we decided to combine a talk and a town meeting at a school. About 300 parents showed up for the talk, and about 70 of them stayed for the town meeting.

Parents are used to talking about personal parenting challenges. The challenge was to help them connect their personal experience to a larger community story and to encourage them to take collective action. At the town meeting, I asked four questions in sequence: "Is this problem we're talking about here—overscheduled kids and underconnected families—only an individual family problem, or is it also a community problem? Are the solutions only individual family solutions, or are they also community solutions? Do you think this community is ready to take action? What actions should we take?"

The first three questions lit the fire: "Yes, it's a community problem! Yes, the solutions must come at the community level as well as the family level! Yes, we're ready to take action!" The meeting became intense as parents worked on the "What shall we do?" question in breakout groups. Afterward, a lot of parents wanted to speak. They were sick of the rat race and eager to do something about it together. One mother stood and said, "I could use something like a Good Housekeeping Seal of Approval for organizations I'm signing my kids up with—something that would show me that this organization will work with me in my efforts to have a balanced family life." That became the seed of an idea eventually adopted by a parent project called Putting Family First (see Chapter 5). On my end, this was my first experience with the power of a public launch event for a citizen therapist project.

There were a couple of moments during the meeting where my clinical skills proved useful. When the discussion started to turn into bashing coaches and community leaders, I intervened like a couples therapist preventing a mutual blame meltdown. "I don't think anybody is setting out to hurt kids," I said, "and I know that there are a lot of competitive pressures on coaches and school leaders. In my view, we're all part of this problem, and we can all be part of the solution." This seemed to connect with most of the parents and later became part of a core theme of the initiative: no villains, no scapegoats.

I did another quick intervention when a woman sitting in the front took a shot at other parents: "This is all well and good, but we're preaching to the choir. It's the parents who aren't here who are the problem." Then somebody added, "There should have been three times as many parents here tonight." As heads nodded, my heart started to sink. But as a family therapist, I know how to intervene when an anxious family member starts pulling the plug on a moment of family courage or connection. I responded, "I think it was Margaret Mead who said that it only takes a small group of committed people to change the world, and indeed that it's never been changed in any other way." After this sank in, I picked up on the choir metaphor: "Every social movement begins with a choir," I said. "And we have a lot of people already in this choir." People sat up in their chairs, and I could sense energy flowing back into the space. Then I brought it home: "If only 12 people with the passion and energy I see in this room had shown up here, I'd have been happy."

More on this project and the FEDS later. For now, we just wanted to give you a sense of how energizing it was for both of us to begin our citizen therapist journeys. Many successes and stumbles later, we wrote this book in hopes of passing on this energy, along with the skills and tools we've learned along the way. Next we define some key terms and then walk you through what this book covers.

WHAT IS A CITIZEN THERAPIST?

Most contemporary therapists understand the connection between personal and public issues. No one could avoid seeing the spillover of public issues during the COVID pandemic of the early 2020s and the political polarization all around us. And of course we are not the first to conceptualize how therapists can contribute at the population level. For example, many therapists work outside of the clinical hour to educate the public about mental health and relational issues. Historically this has taken the form of public speaking, books and magazine articles, and media interviews. In recent years, blogging and developing membership portals have been prominent. A therapist with a clinical specialty in, say, infertility counseling, can reach a large population of people experiencing this challenge. We call such a person a "community educator therapist"—they bring therapeutic knowledge and skills to the wider public, not just clients. It's a valuable way to work upstream from the problems we see in our offices and one that we have engaged in ourselves.

As mentioned earlier, advocacy in the arena of public policy is another way that therapists work to influence the world outside of clinical practice. Much of this is done through professional organizations that prepare therapists with skills in communicating with elected officials and policymakers. For example, many state-level professional associations hold legislative action days when their members lobby state legislators on issues of importance to the profession. Although the focus is generally on the advancement of the profession, therapist advocates can also focus on public policies that directly influence communities in need. In addition to organizational efforts, some therapists are active as individuals in advocating for social-change policies on issues they care deeply about. We call this the "therapist advocate"— a therapist who bring their perspectives and expertise to policymakers. Along with the work of the community educator therapists, advocacy is an important contribution of therapists to the public good. Again, it's an arena in which we have practiced during our careers.

In recent years there has been a renewed interest in *public psychology*; this term originated in the 1960s and received systematic attention culminating in a special issue of the journal *American Psychologist* (Eaton et al., 2021). Most relevant for our purposes is an article by Miles and Fassinger (2021), who called for a scientist–practitioner–advocate model that transcends the traditional two-part scientist–practitioner model by stressing the need to prepare graduate students to become advocates for social justice, particularly in the domain of public policy. Outside the realm of graduate education, our colleague Rob Pasick (2018) has identified for his whole career as a public psychologist, with a remarkable number of projects in which he has promoted institutional change to make psychological services available to new community groups. Thus, there is a term for a public psychologist who advocates for social justice and for expanding clinical services to communities in need.

In light of these existing social-change roles of therapists, why introduce the new term "citizen therapist"? Because the approach described in this book focuses on a kind of activity that has been less common among therapists and other professionals: engaging community members in projects of collective action on health and social problems. The term *citizen therapist* connotes an "alongside of" relationship rather than a service delivery or an "advocating on behalf of" relationship. The citizen therapist's role is that of a catalyst for other citizens (again, defined as people who take responsibility for their communities) to activate their joint capacity for social change. To repeat the key distinction: Citizen therapists (as we conceptualize the role) work with—rather than for—other community members. The short-term outcome of citizen therapist work is a group of everyday people who develop a sense that "we can do important work together for our community." The long-term outcomes of successful projects are visible changes in a specific community and sometimes beyond. The community might be local and geographic, or it might be international via a Web-based group who share the same challenges—or anything in between.

Exhibit 1 offers our way of thinking about three roles of citizen therapists: educator, advocate, and organizer. Although our own work has focused on the organizer role (convening community members to engage in joint projects), we also encourage readers to consider the citizen therapist roles of educator and advocate. Note in Exhibit 1 that we distinguish between the traditional public educator role for therapists, which emphasizes how we bring knowledge to communities, and the citizen therapist educator role, which emphasizes synergy between professional knowledge and knowledge already present in communities. Likewise, we distinguish between traditional advocacy that focuses on either guild interests or influencing public policy on behalf of marginalized communities (both of which are important) and citizen therapist advocacy that collaborates closely with communities working toward policy changes.

Citizen therapists as organizers (again, the focus of this book) are conveners, facilitators, and process leaders for projects that are pressure points for a community. They are catalysts and partners, not managers. They bring interpersonal and group skills to the joint table, along with areas of professional knowledge, and add these to the mix of knowledge and skills that community members bring. At a larger level, citizen therapist work of all kinds is about the role of therapists in reviving democracy defined as the collective agency of "we the diverse people" taking responsibility for solving our collective problems. It's impossible to do citizen therapist work without thinking about democracy all the time.

A final distinction between the citizen therapist role and some other forms of public engagement is that the therapist can engage with any community struggling with a pressing concern, including but not confined to communities that have been disenfranchised. The "we the people" in a citizen therapist project can be a largely upper-middle-class White community struggling with the social pathologies of contemporary family life (see Chapter 5) or a largely low-income urban-dwelling American Indian community struggling with the impact of diabetes (see Chapter 2). With no political or ideological litmus tests for who comes to the table to create a project, it can involve police

EXHIBIT 1. Three Roles for Citizen Therapists

1. Educator
   - Mission: Capacity building for a democratic way of life. Equipping people with the knowledge and tools for decision making, self-care, close relationships, participation in community—and less dependence on professionals
   - Practice: Democratic knowledge sharing. Blending professional expertise and community expertise, with special emphasis on sharing the knowledge and wisdom of community members
   - Difference from traditional educator role: Not hierarchical and expert-oriented, two-way learning (everyone a teacher and learner), valuing local knowledge and not just universal, academic knowledge
   - Examples: Community education that accesses parents' knowledge and energy; a public health education campaign on lead risk to children carried out by a group of professionals and community members; using Web 2.0 in a way that engages public reflection and deliberation

2. Advocate
   - Mission: Open up public resources and influence public policy. An emphasis on policies and resources that develop capacity for personal and community agency instead of consumer dependence
   - Practice: Joint education, persuasion, and pressure. Working closely with other community members to influence public leaders to provide more equitable distribution of resources and to adopt policies that engage citizens in personal and public problem solving
   - Difference from traditional advocate role: Not professional guild oriented, always teamed with other citizens, emphasizes the role of government as partner and capacity builder, not parent
   - Example: Neighborhood advocates persuading the City of Seattle to create a collaborative neighborhood design within its comprehensive city planning

3. Organizer
   - Mission: Community-based problem solving. Activating and partnering with grassroots groups of citizens to tackle community pressure points
   - Practice: Community organizing. Democratic planning, leadership development, outreach, and action initiatives that call upon the talents and passions of a specific community
   - Difference from traditional community organizer: Involves an important role for professionals, willing to use academic knowledge "on tap," not "on top"
   - Examples: Citizen health care projects described in this book

officers and Black community members who feel oppressed by the police (see Chapter 9). Political conservatives can engage with liberals without the citizen therapist asking anyone to embrace contemporary social justice perspectives (see Chapter 10). We deal with diversity and social justice by creating containers within which people who differ along the lines of power and race come together in flattened hierarchies to solve problems that they cannot without each other.

We know that the citizen therapist concept can be hard to grasp at first. That's why this book is full of project examples of our work and that of other therapists. As you read the stories, we encourage you to identify your clinical passions or personal or family challenges and then imagine the communities of people who face a similar health or social challenge. In other words, place problems you care about in the context of a large number of people sharing the same concern. Then connect their concerns to a larger picture that might include issues such as social isolation or lack of public understanding. In other words, identify the bigger landscape that these clients navigate and then conceive some initial ideas about how they could do two things: better navigate that landscape together and eventually change features of that landscape. Mutual support and social change: This combination is the sweet spot for citizen therapist activities as we think of them. And as we emphasize repeatedly in this book, citizen therapists continue in their day jobs of providing therapeutic services to clients. Just as the citizen legislator serves in a state legislature in addition to their regular paid work in their home communities, citizen therapists approach this work as their contributions to the public good in addition to their everyday work as healers.

A note about realistic expectations: There are times in life when active engagement in community work is feasible and energizing and other times when it would cause overload. In this book we are more interested in planting a way of thinking in the minds of readers so that when the time is right, they have some guideposts to become active in their communities. Sometimes it's enough to just incubate an idea and talk to others about it, with no expectation of near-term action. We know a therapist living with chronic illness who is inspired by the ideas we present in this book and is waiting for a time when her energy level permits her to start a project that would be different from anything she sees going on in disability communities. For everything there is a season. Having said that, we believe that therapists who can take the plunge into this kind of civic work will reap personal and professional rewards. We certainly have.

OVERVIEW OF THE BOOK

We've written this book with three main audiences in mind. First is graduate students and new professionals in the therapy field who are interested in making a difference in the world beyond their clinical work. Building in time and space for citizen therapist work at the outset of one's career may be easier than doing so after making commitments that might have to be curtailed to do this kind of work. The second audience is retired therapists who have the time and energy for engaging in civic work. The third set of readers is experienced therapists who are itching to get involved in public work and might consider shuffling their current priorities to make room for it. Although one of the projects described in Chapter 10 is in Africa, this book focuses primarily on the U.S. context, including its democracy, which, although currently under strain, allows for citizen engagement in civic and institutional systems.

Chapter 1 completes Part I, our overview of citizen therapist work, by presenting its theoretical framework. Therein we describe the origins of our framework in Boyte and colleagues' public work model as we've adapted it to our citizen health care model.

Part II (Chapters 2–4) describes citizen therapist projects in health care: around diabetes (Chapter 2 on the Family Education Diabetes Series, our longest-standing project), on smoking cessation in a Job Corps setting (Chapter 3), and in a clinic-wide community building (Chapter 4).

Part III (Chapters 5–7) describes our work in cultural change. Two projects involve parents: Chapter 5 (Putting Family First) addresses challenges particularly pertinent to parents in middle-class families in hypercompetitive communities and Chapter 6 (Citizen Father Project) involves low-income, unmarried single fathers giving back to their community. Chapter 7 (Braver Angels) tells the story of a project on political polarization—couples therapy on a national scale.

Part IV has two chapters on projects dealing with race: the Relationships Project with young Black men in a public high school (Chapter 8) and the Police and Black Men Project (Chapter 9). The focus of both projects is on agency and building empowered relationships across differences, rather than an us-versus-them approach.

Part V includes chapters addressing how to become a citizen therapist and how to succeed in this work. Chapter 10 profiles several projects of other citizen therapists and discusses core elements of their work. Chapter 11 describes how to maintain collaborative projects over a long period. Chapter 12 offers ideas on how to get projects funded and how to evaluate them. Chapter 13 drills down on how to get started in citizen therapist work, including how to find an issue and a community and how to exercise process leadership. We also discuss lessons we learned from projects that failed to get traction. Chapter 14 addresses the citizen therapist as a person and professional, including the self of the therapist and different roles such as graduate student, community therapist, academic, and retired therapist. The afterword is a call to action and offers an important resource for readers who want to go further with this kind of work.

We have some advice for how to read this book. Start with Chapter 1 on foundations of our model, sample the chapters in Parts II through IV depending on your interest in the various issues addressed in the projects, and then focus on the Part V chapters to integrate your understanding of citizen therapist work and learn how to get started.

Here is how we envision what therapists can contribute to a troubled world. The cornerstone is that therapists believe in human agency and the capacity for constructive change. The world needs this belief and related skills to renew our civic life. This renewal of our commonwealth won't come just from clinical work in the personal sphere or from supporting the right candidates in the public sphere. We can create a new breed of public actor with exceptional interpersonal skills: citizen therapists for a troubled world.

1   FOUNDATIONS OF CITIZEN THERAPIST WORK

Psychotherapy appears to be the quintessentially private profession. People go to therapists for personal problems, not to complain about society or politics, and therapists enter the profession because they are drawn to intimate psychological dialogue. Therapy involves tighter rules about dual relationships than do most other professions: We relate to clients in the office but generally not in the community. Thus, it seems like a big leap to think of therapists as public citizens engaging in community building and social change. We might help our clients engage in their own communities, and we might do the same ourselves as volunteers or private citizens. But community engagement has not been in the professional wheelhouse of therapists. And the role of the therapist in sustaining democracy—well, that's rarely discussed.

This chapter begins with the public role of therapists, including false dichotomies and problematic assumptions that have hindered this role, followed by a presentation of the idea of the "citizen professional." We then describe our own model of citizen therapist work, which we call "citizen health care."

https://doi.org/10.1037/0000378-002
Becoming a Citizen Therapist: Integrating Community Problem-Solving Into Your Work as a Healer, by W. J. Doherty and T. J. Mendenhall

IDEAS THAT STAND IN THE WAY OF A PUBLIC ROLE FOR THERAPISTS[1]

All of the therapeutic professions—psychiatry, psychology, clinical social work, marriage and family therapy, psychiatric nursing, professional counseling—share assumptions about the nature of professional practice that emerged in the early 20th century (Sullivan, 2004). As Brint and Levy (1999) found in their historical research on contemporary professions, until the 1930s professional leaders often articulated larger visions of making contributions to the public good and building a democratic nation. In subsequent decades of the 20th century, most professions focused on guild interests and did their public service through committees and task forces created to educate the public or advocate for public policies. Although in recent decades there has been a revival of focus on the public mission of fields such as psychology (e.g., Eaton et al., 2021, on "public psychology"), the primary emphasis for therapists has been on how we work with individual clients to understand and counteract toxic social influences such as racism (Comas-Díaz, 2020; Lee, 2013, 2018). Largely missing has been articulated models for therapists to be public actors engaging with communities.

Before talking about models for engaging with communities, however, we begin by describing some of the misguided assumptions and beliefs that we believe have inhibited the development of publicly engaged therapists.

False Dichotomies That Shape Therapy's Paradigm

First is the private–public split, the notion that some problems are purely private and others purely public. (By *public*, we mean larger social, cultural, economic, political, and environmental spheres.) For example, depression in the therapy literature appears almost exclusively as a private problem—depending on your orientation, either a chemical imbalance or a psychological disorder or both. Widespread poverty, on the other hand, is seen as a public problem, with societal and economic origins. In teaching and research, we generally overlook how depression and poverty mutually influence each other—for example, how poverty leads to depression and how depression keeps people mired in poverty (Ridley et al., 2020). Or take schizophrenia,

---

[1]This section is adapted from "Families and Therapists as Citizens: The Families and Democracy Project," by W. J. Doherty and J. S. Carroll, in E. Aldarondo (Ed.), *Advancing Social Justice Through Clinical Practice* (pp. 223–244), 2007, Taylor & Francis. Copyright 2007 by Taylor & Francis. Adapted with permission.

a prototypically individual medical disorder that often is treated—or not treated—in jails and prisons, which have become the de facto mental health system for many people with serious and persistent mental illness (Kuehn, 2014). Mental illness, then, is a public problem, not just a private one, but the discourse of professional psychotherapy tends to concentrate only on the private domain, leaving the public domain to public health specialists and policymakers. Although it could be argued that clinical social work has a stronger community perspective than do other mental health professions, the everyday practice of clinical social workers seems not very different from that of other therapists, despite critiques from within social work about its neglect of a larger societal orientation (McLaughlin, 2002).

The second dichotomy is provider–consumer roles. This duality runs deep in contemporary American culture (Boyte & Kari, 1996; Cohen, 2008; Doherty, 2022). Individuals are either the provider of a service or the recipient of a service, the former the seller and the latter the buyer. Professional providers are experts on the problems of consumer clients, and consumers are assumed to be concerned only with getting the best service for themselves as individuals, not with anything related to the common good of a community. Our concern here is not with legitimate differences in roles or with the notion of therapist expertise but with how the service provider role has come to dominate the way we think about the work of therapists and other professionals. Missing from this discourse is a way to think of ourselves as citizens, not just providers, and as community members engaged in partnerships with other citizens to tackle the public problems that show up in our offices and clinics. Also missing is the idea of our clients as citizens with something to contribute to their communities beyond the idea that when clients function better personally, they will be better citizens. The provider–consumer dichotomy leaves out a third alternative—civic partnerships in which we are neither providers nor consumers—the kind of civic engagement that our world sorely needs in an era of widespread disengagement from public life (Putnam, 2001, 2020).

The third dichotomy is personal therapy versus community work. By personal therapy, we mean work with individuals, families, or small groups, as distinguished from community-based activities for larger groups. As Sullivan (2004) observed, U.S. professions since the 1920s have divided themselves into the vast majority of providers who work in the individual sphere and a minority who work in the public sphere. (The same split occurs to varying degrees in other countries.) Examples are clinical medicine versus public health medicine, clinical nursing versus public health nursing, clinical social work versus community social work, and clinical or counseling psychology versus community psychology. When leaders in a profession want more emphasis on the public realm, they generally spin off a new subspecialty. In most cases, that community specialty then becomes marginalized from the mainstream of the profession that spawned it (Albee, 1998). Social work is the main exception, but in that case it's clinical work that is disparaged in academic programs that prioritize community work as the core of the profession (McLaughlin, 2002). And it's important to note that in psychology there are a number of clinical-community psychology graduate programs.

Despite recent efforts in areas such as public psychology (Miles & Fassinger, 2021) and critical social work (C. Brown, 2021), the dichotomy mainly holds: Therapists and community professionals are cut off from meaningful interactions with each other. They read different books and articles, they attend different meetings, and they rely on different sources of knowledge. In our own work to transcend this dichotomy, we promote the idea that therapists can engage in community work while keeping their day jobs doing therapy. They would do this work in partnership with other community members and sometimes with professionals who do community work as their main focus.

The three dichotomies we've identified run deep in the paradigm of psychotherapy. They keep us away from civic engagement, leaving it to personal volunteer work not integrated with our professional identities—a lack of integration characterizing most modern professions and the basis of calls for the development of "citizen professionalism" (Boyte et al., 2018; Dzur, 2017). We want to emphasize that the idea of the citizen therapist is not mainly a call for therapists to do more for their communities. It's a part of a reenvisioning of what it means to be a professional in modern democracies.

Conventional Beliefs That Limit Us

The beliefs we now turn to don't keep us off the playing field of public work, but they limit our scope and effectiveness. We don't claim that all therapists hold these beliefs, but we see them as quite pervasive.

Community work is for low-income communities. The assumption here is that only low-income communities are in need of community-based initiatives, as if well-to-do suburbs are not also suffering from a lack of social capital and civic spirit. The upshot is that if a therapist does not have access to an inner city or a poor rural community, there is nothing meaningful to do except to write a check to nonprofits that work with needy communities. A more accurate belief, in our view, is that all communities can benefit from the collective work of citizens to tackle local problems that often have broader implications.

Collaborating with organizations is the same thing as working with communities. Doherty and Beaton (2000) made a distinction between *community systems* (organized institutions, programs, and agencies) and *communities* (groups of individuals and families that have interlocking relationships and a degree of shared culture and purpose). There are a number of models of collaboration between therapists and community institutions for the benefit of clients (Imber-Black, 1988; McDaniel et al., 2014) but fewer models showing therapists how to work directly with communities themselves. In our observation, many therapists equate community work with talking with social service professionals about common clients.

A therapist's social responsibility can be adequately addressed through pro bono clinical services. As helpful as donated service is for those who cannot afford treatment, it does not transcend the split between individual work and community work. Even when organized by professional associations, say, after a disaster, pro bono therapy offers an important public good but does not alter the fundamental private–public dichotomy in the profession.

Students should first master clinical skills before getting involved in community work. This belief assumes that a therapist is fundamentally a service provider to individuals and that the public work is an add-on. The same mistake was made decades ago by medical schools that taught anatomy and physiology, including dissecting cadavers, before they taught students how to interact humanely with actual patients. The template for professional identity is set from the first day of training. For medicine it was an identity as an applied biologist. For those of us therapists (like Bill) who came to a public perspective later in our careers, it is tempting to see our own developmental path (clinical focus for many years, then community involvement) as a necessary sequence for the next generation. But just as a medical student can embrace a humanistic, biopsychosocial model from their first day in medical school, so too can a therapy student develop, from the start, an identity as both a personal healer and a community actor.

Public policy advocacy is the primary way that professionals can make a difference in the public realm. Professionals who see the limitations of clinical work for social change often assume that the only alternative is public policy advocacy. Although advocacy is essential to the public contributions of a profession and, we believe, can be done in a citizen therapist way (see the introduction to this book), traditional advocacy approaches have several downsides and limitations as the primary focus of public action by professionals. We outline these here:

- If not done in partnership with communities, advocacy can take the form of professional elites talking to political elites about the needs of nonelite people.

- Traditional public advocacy often does not call on the resources of communities, focusing instead on outside resources and unintentionally communicating the idea that the local community is barren of resources. In our citizen health care work, we always pair a "needs" question with a question about the existing community resources that can be activated.

- Advocacy generally does not engage communities in tackling questions of larger meaning and collective action, focusing instead on specific programs, technical policies, and complex legislation. The more technical the policy, the less involved regular people are likely to be.

- Advocacy can be ineffective when viewed by policymakers as predictable, partisan, or guild promoting—characteristics often true of professional advocacy efforts. In terms of engagement with elected officials, we admire the approach of our colleague Karen Bogenschneider (2023), who stresses building relationships with legislators and policymakers on both sides of the political aisle, bringing research knowledge to policy topics, and avoiding coming across as predictable and one-sided.

To be clear, we believe that public policy advocacy has a useful role in social change, and we've done our share of it. But it is a selectively powerful tool, mostly practiced well by professionals trained to work in partisan political systems, and not the main way to engage a broad range of therapists in community action. Most of all, our concern is the assumption that public engagement by therapists is equivalent to public policy advocacy.

Being socially responsible requires taking liberal–left political positions. Most therapy organizations that engage issues of social responsibility appear to come from a liberal–left political stance (Redding, 2001). We are concerned about the underlying message this sends to therapists of other political views and to community members we might partner with that citizen therapy work is inherently liberal or progressive. In a politically pluralistic society, if public work by therapists requires adherence to one subset of political views, then it will always have limited potential for engaging many communities. Our own work described in this book has no political litmus tests for participants and has been supported by people from divergent political persuasions.

THE CITIZEN PROFESSIONAL IDEA

Although this book focuses on the citizen role of therapists, we want to reemphasize that this idea is part of a larger movement toward reevaluating the role of professionals in democratic societies (Boyte, 2004; Dzur, 2008). (That is why we sometimes use the broader term *citizen professional*.) It emphasizes how professionals of all kinds (law, medicine, architecture, etc.)

can contribute to the civic life of communities while also playing their traditional role in providing specialized services. It challenges the 20th-century view of the professional as a detached expert who may critique social systems but does not work to change those systems and who, most importantly, sees communities in terms of their needs for professional and societal help but not their capacities for collective, transformative action. In the same vein, traditional professional ethics codes emphasize the expertise and benevolence of the professional serving clients, but these codes render invisible the roles of professionals as citizens of a broader community. Following are essential elements of citizen professionalism as we envision it.

Citizen professionalism is an identity: seeing oneself first as a citizen with special expertise working alongside other citizens with their own special expertise to solve community problems that require everyone's effort. (Again, the citizen concept here refers not to legal status but to being a stakeholder in a community and society.) This is not just an idealistic self-image but a grounded realization that the really big problems in health care, education, and social welfare—sometimes known as "wicked problems"—cannot be solved by professionals working alone, nor by government action alone. We will not make headway against the tide unless we all row together.

Citizen professionals have a body of knowledge about the connections between the personal and the public dimensions of their professional practice. Citizen physicians, for example, understand the connection between diabetes, the fast-food industry, and cultural practices of diet and exercise. Citizen lawyers who work on divorce understand how the adversarial legal system undermines the ability of couples with children to find cooperative ways to end their relationship and build a different kind of family going forward. Citizen therapists understand how societal and cultural forces such as isolation, inequality, and stigmatization create conditions for mental illness and relational problems.

Citizen professionals have a set of skills for facilitating public conversations and catalyzing public action. They are able to bring together other citizens for public conversations and local action projects to address community needs. Citizen parent educators, for example, have the skills to lead parents in a discussion that connects children's safety and the social cohesion of neighborhoods, to encourage parents to become active in their communities around issues of safety, and to create a venue where parents can meet with community leaders to get involved. This book articulates a set of public skills for therapists.

When it comes to research, citizen professionals have access to the rich tradition of community-based participatory research (also called action research and participatory action research). This approach involves close collaborations between the researcher and a community of other citizens in every stage of the project, from identifying the problem to designing interventions to evaluating the outcomes. It features a democratic process in which everyone's expertise is brought to bear (Brush et al. 2020).

There is an important distinction between this idea of the citizen professional and specialized forms of full-time community practice. Citizen professionals as defined here have their primary base in service delivery. They are grounded in patient care, education, therapy, social service, and other forms of personal practice. (In our experience, this kind of intensive personal engagement with clients can create social trust that opens the door to collaborative community projects.) Our vision in this book is the renewal of frontline professional practice by therapists as involving a dimension of work alongside other citizens—not as an alternative to clinical practice but as a rich addition in which personal healing and community engagement are integrated into the identity of a citizen therapist.

ORIGINS OF THE CITIZEN THERAPIST MODEL

The citizen therapist idea is not confined to one theoretical or practice model. We welcome our colleagues to develop their own approaches (see Chapter 10 for examples). However, the DNA of the citizen therapist role as we envision it involves the therapist helping to create opportunities for citizens to work together to solve health and social problems. To repeat: It's distinct from therapists volunteering in their communities or bringing their clinical expertise to groups outside of their practice. Another point of emphasis is that citizen therapist work involves developing a set of skills (having a model, if you will) in public engagement, just as all forms of psychotherapy require a skill base. It's a disciplined practice developed over time rather than just a set of activities in community—just as, to use a clinical analogy, family therapy is more than simply meeting with a client's family.

Our own citizen therapist model has gone by two names, depending on the context of the work: citizen health care and the families and democracy model. We started out with the latter but then, after realizing that in health care, grouping the terms *family* and *democracy* did not compute, we switched to *citizen health care*. Even though many of our projects are outside of health care, for the sake of simplicity in this book we use citizen health care for our framework, thinking of health in its broadest sense. We offer this model as one way to do citizen therapist work, and we welcome more frameworks from others.

Our framework grew out of the public work model of the Center for Democracy and Citizenship at the University of Minnesota, as developed by Harry Boyte, Nancy Kari, Nancy Shelton, and their colleagues (Boyte & Kari, 1996; Boyte et al., 2000). Boyte, a political theorist who was schooled in the civil rights struggles of the 1960s and the Saul Alinsky tradition of community organizing, moved from a radical-left political philosophy in the 1970s to what he called a "new populism" in the 1980s and 1990s. The public work model has three main orienting ideas:

- *Human beings as producers or cocreators of the world.* Public work is defined as sustained, visible, serious effort by a diverse mix of ordinary people that creates things of lasting civic or public significance. This is a citizen dynamic in contrast to the pervasive provider–consumer dynamic of American culture.

- *The importance of public life.* A public life is essential for human flourishing. The privatization of contemporary life undermines well-being and leads to the unhealthy dominance of impersonal forces such as the marketplace over human affairs.

- *Democratic, relational power.* Through exercising "civic muscle," ordinary people can influence the world of institutions, professions, and the marketplace. Democracy is not confined to voting and volunteering as a private citizen; it's about joint efforts with other citizens to build a robust public world. This is more a politics of collaborative relationships for solving public problems than the traditional politics of petition and protest.

Since the late 1990s, we have been applying this framework to our citizen therapist work across a range of populations and settings, and we have articulated the theory and skills behind this work under the rubric of citizen health care. (A list of projects and populations can be found at https://www.citizenprofessional.org.)

OVERVIEW OF THE CITIZEN HEALTH CARE MODEL

Given its origins as we just described, our model stresses the importance of civic engagement to strengthen personal health and social well-being, the need to transcend the traditional provider–consumer model of health care and professional service delivery, and a vision of ordinary citizens creating public initiatives in partnership with therapists and other professionals. The main principle is that the greatest untapped resource for improving health and social well-being is the knowledge, wisdom, and lived experience of individuals, families, communities who have faced challenging issues in their everyday lives. This principle is worth reading a couple of times. With professional resources often being tapped out, there is a huge underaccessed resource in the energy and investment of people who have "been there"— they have experienced life challenges and have contributions to make to meet those challenges in their communities.

In practice, this principle means that the first people we approach as partners in projects are individuals who have lived with and coped well with a health or social problem and who are ready to give back. They know diabetes or single fathering or overscheduled kids from the inside, and they've found ways to manage and succeed. We offer them ways to organize together and make a difference for others. In our projects, we usually operationalize the term *community* as people who have faced challenges, who are now above water, and who are open to organizing in order to address these challenges in a larger way.

The other core principles are as follows:

- People must be engaged as producers and contributors to their communities and not just as clients or consumers of services.

- Therapists and other professionals can play an important role in initiatives when they learn to partner with other citizens in identifying challenges, mobilizing resources, generating plans, and carrying out public actions.

- If you begin with an established program, you will not end up with an initiative that is owned and operated by citizens. But a citizen initiative might create or adopt a program as one of its activities.

- A local community becomes energized when it retrieves its own historical, cultural, and religious traditions and brings these to bear on a current goal or problem.

- Initiatives should have a bold vision (a BHAG—a big, hairy, audacious goal) while working pragmatically on focused, specific goals.

In addition to these core principles, citizen health care involves implementation strategies. These strategies help avoid the ever-present risk of lapsing into a traditional program and professional service models as well as the typical volunteer approach that invites people to be helpers but not creators and producers. You will see the following strategies (and the principles behind them) played out in the projects described in this book.

- Employ democratic planning and decision making at every step.
- Emphasize mutual teaching and learning between professionals and community members.

- Create ways to fold new learnings back into the community.
- Continually identify and develop new leaders.
- Use professional expertise selectively—"on tap," not "on top."
- Generate public visibility through media and community events.
- Forge a sense of larger purpose beyond helping immediate participants.

We want to highlight the importance of developing new leaders as something that was not as clear to us at the outset of our citizen therapist work. Everyone's job is to look for people to join the initiative, to add to its energy and resources, and eventually to become leaders. Otherwise, the first round of leaders will get tired, begin to act entitled, or become rigid. For projects that are planned to exist over a number of years, we now believe that it takes three generations of leaders for an initiative to become mature: the original visioning and planning group, the next wave of participants who come on board to lead action initiatives, and then those who come originally to participate in activities in a fully established program and who then move into leadership. Having said that, some projects with more time-focused goals do not require multiple generations of leaders.

A final note that will become clearer as we describe projects: The most enduring projects (going through multiple generations of citizen leaders) tend to be housed in institutions that have access to a pool of clients or participants and that see this work as part of their mission. In those settings, getting institutional buy-in from administrators and staff is a necessary first step, and some staff are involved in the projects where they learn to be citizen professionals. However, the projects always emphasize the cocreative work of lay leaders (ordinary citizens) whose first loyalties are to their community and not to an institution.

After more than 2 decades into our own learning curves in citizen therapist work, we can attest to the joy and enrichment we've experienced. We have no sense of helplessness in the face of mounting social problems and polarization in our country and world. Public stressors, if anything, have increased since we began this journey as citizen therapists. But we feel like we are in the fray, in the struggle to make a better world. We are in this struggle as therapists who know something about human relationships, not as social critics standing above and pointing fingers at the wrong side or as partisans wishing that our political party would solve the nation's woes by decisive victories at the polls. The problems run deeper. They are in the social fabric of anxiety, distrust, inequality, and isolation. For too long, therapists have stayed in our offices with highly developed personal skills and underdeveloped public skills. We can do more. The next set of chapters details some of our efforts to do more.

PART II HEALTH CARE PROJECTS

2

THE FAMILY EDUCATION DIABETES SERIES

Tackling the Diabetes Epidemic in an American Indian Community

The project described in this chapter is a health promotion initiative cocreated through the efforts of medical and mental health professionals and Elders and leaders in the Minneapolis/Saint Paul American Indian[1] community. The Family Education Diabetes Series (FEDS) engages low-income, urban-dwelling American Indians and their families in an active forum of fellowship and support that combines contemporary knowledge about disease management and purposeful efforts to reclaim Native foods, activities, and cultures. Guided by the citizen health care model, the group from the outset embraced the premise that everyone involved has something valuable to contribute to a collective effort to address an ominous health threat.

As the longest standing, most established, and most thoroughly evaluated project that we have worked on, a considerable number of publications are already available that tell the story of the FEDS, including its evolution and outcome data (Berge et al., 2009; Mendenhall, 2021; Mendenhall et al., 2010, 2012, 2018). A special focus of the following description is on how

---

[1]We use the terms *American Indian*, *Indigenous*, and *Native* interchangeably. This is consistent with preferences of Elders in the FEDS.

https://doi.org/10.1037/0000378-003
Becoming a Citizen Therapist: Integrating Community Problem-Solving Into Your Work as a Healer, by W. J. Doherty and T. J. Mendenhall

health improvement efforts are integrated with community members' reclamation of cherished Indigenous traditions of "walking in balance."

ORIGIN OF THE FEDS

The FEDS evolved as an offshoot of the Partners in Diabetes project described in the introduction to this book. Nan LittleWalker and Betty GreenCrow, both well-respected local Native Elders, were support partners in Partners in Diabetes, but they maintained that most Native people living with diabetes would never benefit from it. They made clear to us that the majority of their community did not trust Western medical providers (and usually with good reason, based on disrespectful and racist wrongdoings over generations). They explained, too, that most did not carry health insurance or have adequate funds to cover copays for health visits, which further prevented opportunities to talk with other patients or spouses in the clinic-based Partners in Diabetes program. And finally, Nan and Betty maintained that much of the training and information included in Partners in Diabetes was relatively generic in nature, thereby not aligning with Native customs and viewpoints about health that would tap Indigenous wisdom.

I (Tai) and a physician colleague began a 3-year-long conversation with Nan and Betty, during which time I got out of the comfort zone of my own turf (the medical clinic). In the basement of a small church housing the Interfaith Action of Greater Saint Paul's Department of Indian Work (DIW), surrounded by Native art, images, quilts, drums, and other musical instruments, Nan, Betty, and other Elders taught me about the diversity of Indigenous tribes' beliefs regarding health, the Medicine Wheel, and walking in balance. I learned about how generations of colonization, forced relocation, poverty, processed foods, and lost ways of life have disrupted this balance, with devastating health consequences. I was invited to local powwows and community events and took part in talking circles focused on how Native ways could be reclaimed toward healthy living in combination with medical knowledge about diabetes management. I learned the value of prayer, smudging (burning sweet grass or sage), and spirit plates in local meetings. Along the way, Elders learned from me about how the culture of Western medicine and research universities is driven by relative value units, evidence-based practices, peer-reviewed articles, and never-ending searches for research funding. This helped the Elders better understand the context and struggles of health providers who otherwise appeared like rushed and data-obsessed workaholics.

It was through this reciprocal learning and trust building that the Family Education Diabetes Series was ultimately created. It began with an acronym, the FEDS, originally suggested by Nan and Betty as a remembrance of the genocide of Native peoples. The U.S. federal government, whose agents are colloquially referred to as "the feds" (in lowercase), was a colonizer. In that light, Nan and Betty thought that it was empowering to call ourselves the FEDS (in capital letters). I was initially worried that this could work against our group in terms of community optics and future efforts to seek funds for program evaluation, but I was wrong. The name stuck, and the initiative flourished.

Since 2001, the FEDS has met biweekly—mostly in that same church basement (meetings went online during the COVID-19 pandemic, and more recently, in-person gatherings resumed at a different community site). The program is advertised via word of mouth in the local community, and participants include American Indian patients, loved ones, former-participants-turned-mentors, medical and mental health providers, health researchers, students (undergraduate, graduate), and tribal Elders. Some participants have consistently taken part in the FEDS since its inception; some come for one or two series (described below); others come for specific sessions that target specific topics; and some come intermittently as they are able to or interested.

PROGRAM CONTENT AND PROCESSES

The FEDS functions as a health program that engages low-income, urban-dwelling American Indians and their families in an active forum of education, fellowship, and support. Each program series (the *S* in FEDS) includes 16 biweekly sessions, followed by a 3- to 4-week break before picking back up again. Participants consist of new participants who either have diabetes or are recognized to be at high risk for it (about 10–15 people) and their family members; mentors (about 10–15 American Indians who participated in previous FEDS programs); medical and behavioral health providers, including researchers (4–5) and students (2–10); and tribal Elders (2–4). As participants arrive, they collect individualized folders that contain health data recorded at previous visits (or a new folder for first-timers). Mentors, providers, and students conduct foot checks and record each participant's weight and body mass index, blood pressure, and blood sugar in the folders. Providers track their own personal data as well (everyone involved, regardless of role, is invested in their own and each other's health). Professional and community participants visit with each other in pairs or small groups throughout this time.

Evening events formally begin with one of our Elders leading the group in a prayer, during which thanks is given for our collective commitment to the FEDS' mission, and guidance from the Creator (however defined) is requested so that we may be successful in our work together. A spirit plate (containing samples of each ingredient of our evening's food) is sanctified and then shared outdoors with Ancestors who are believed to be watching over us. Each participant is then blessed through smudging (via burning sweet grass or sage) as a way to welcome good life forces and healing energy to our forum.

Meals consistent with American Indian cultures are then shared communally, along with discussions led by a Native cook about how they were prepared, indicated portion sizes, and costs. An educational forum ensues (the *E* in FEDS). This takes place in talking circles, small- and large-group discussions, and a variety of lively activities (e.g., traditional music, dancing and aerobics, impromptu theater and role plays). We always make sure to include both up-to-date clinical information (usually via one of our own providers, researchers, or an invited guest speaker) and wisdom from lived experience (usually via one of our own mentors, Elders, or an invited community member). For example, copresenters may talk about the physiological benefits of physical activity, paired with advice about how to do this while living in a neighborhood that does not feel safe (e.g., chair aerobics at home, power walking at a local mall). They may share contemporary knowledge about how metabolic functioning impacts serotonin production in the brain in a conversation about depression, alongside culturally sensitive ways to talk about or seek help for mental health needs. All told, series topics are remarkably diverse (see the examples in Exhibit 2.1), and no two series are exactly the same because the program forever evolves in response to the feedback, interests, contributions, and engagement of professional and community members who are involved. FEDS evenings conclude with time for more informal sharing and support. Sessions are scheduled for 3 hours, but most participants arrive early and stay late, and some stay even later to help wash dishes, clean the kitchen, and reorganize the space (chairs, tables, program supplies).

WHAT THE FEDS IS AND WHAT IT IS NOT

Citizen health care groups such as the FEDS function somewhere in the middle of a continuum where on one end professional experts are the drivers (the traditional medical model) and on the other end lay community members

EXHIBIT 2.1. Examples of FEDS Session Topics

- Introduction: Diabetes as a Disease and Diabetes in the American Indian Community
- Dietary Guidelines and Portion Sizes
- Exercise and Physical Activity
- Obesity and Weight Control
- Living With a Chronic Illness
- Blood Glucose Monitoring and Control
- Diabetes and Eye Diseases/Retinopathy
- Blood Pressure and Cholesterol
- Heart Disease and Stroke
- Stress Management and Strategies
- Foot Care and Wound Care
- Medical Services and Supplies
- Depression and Anxiety
- Working With Your Doctors
- Sticking With It: Staying Motivated and Family/Social Support
- Review: Putting It All Together

lead without professional involvement (as in Alcoholics Anonymous). In diabetes care, the first model would include a mobile diabetes clinic, and the second could be a peer support group. Each is a familiar model and would be easier to pull off than a citizen health care group that involves both patients and professionals in partnership. In the FEDS, professional expertise is "on tap," not "on top," and patient and family knowledge permeates everything we do. In alignment with Medicine Wheel notions of walking in balance that honor the mind, body, spirit, and community, we work to simultaneously balance professionals' and lay members' contributions.

The FEDS is not a fee-for-service program wherein community members can come receive health care interventions or personalized advice about their diabetes. However, presenters do encourage participants to follow up with their doctor (if they have one) for such counsel, and they help participants identify accessible care with local culturally competent providers. At the same time, the FEDS is more than a social support program. Although the content discussed is always framed within Indigenous traditions, it is explicitly paired with contemporary research and knowledge gained through Western medicine that inform good disease management. Most of the providers involved in the FEDS are not Native, yet they participate actively in the initiative's programming.

Although the FEDS often has grant funding, it has not required external funding to survive. It is owned and operated by its citizens, and they work together to ensure continuity. In fact, the FEDS' sustainability for 20-plus years across both stout and lean times represents one its most notable successes. I (Tai) and others have worked with Native Elders and agency leaders in the DIW to secure research grants to support program evaluation. Similarly, our Elders and agency leaders have worked to get resource grants to cover testing provisions, food, and other program supplies. When we have funding, we have access to greater varieties of food, more rigorous metabolic testing and data tracking, formal research assistants, and honoraria for outside speakers. When we do not have funding, participants contribute food, potluck style, and professionals volunteer their time to speak or analyze data. When the program's supporting organization recently restructured and the FEDS' church basement was no longer available, alternative gathering sites were found. When COVID-19 prevented in-person gatherings, professional and lay citizens worked together to purchase necessary technologies like Zoom and then taught participants how to use them). One way or another, with and without funding, the program lives on.

IMPACT AND FOLLOW-UP

During FEDS' early days, it was enough to "sell" the program to my (Tai's) university supervisors and the DIW administrators by way of its innovative merits alone. This new idea—pairing professional expertise with the lived experience and wisdom of Native people who are working to reclaim Indigenous traditions toward improved health—had enough face validity to allow for some professional and resource risks. Furthermore, the 3 years of meetings and trust-building efforts between me, my physician colleague, and several community Elders who informed the program's creation represented a persuasive foundation to try it out. And the FEDS did, indeed, appear to work for its early participants, per their anecdotal and informal accounts.

It did not take long, however, before external stakeholders began to ask for data showing outcomes and effectiveness. Because we were already collecting health data from the very beginning (good disease management requires this!), moving forward with formal testing of the FEDS was a logical and relatively easy next step. Evaluation has been ongoing, including weight, body mass index, systolic and diastolic blood pressure, random blood glucose, and average metabolic control (A1C). New FEDS participants consistently show improvement across these parameters (e.g., a mean of 20 pounds of weight loss in 1 year), and veteran participants evidence either further improvement or sustained change (maintained weight loss for > 3 years). Formal assessments of disease-related knowledge are also administered in pre–post successions, and these too yield positive results. Qualitative interviews conducted in the contexts of talking circles indicate that family and social support are key ingredients toward positive health change (Mendenhall et al., 2012, 2018; Seal et al., 2016).

Evaluations of the FEDS will continue, with or without external funding, across new cohorts of program participants. These are conducted through single-group, repeated-measures designs—not randomized controlled trials—because all community members are welcome to participate. Elders long ago steered us away from having control groups who would be denied the program. The FEDS belongs to its community, to everyone and at any time. Competitiveness for external funding has not been weakened by this decision. Instead, it has served as grounds for supporting work as community owned, even "community cherished."

SPIN-OFF PROJECTS

Several projects described in this book demonstrate how new citizen health care projects evolve as offshoots from their earlier ones. In the FEDS, this has happened in two exciting ways.

First, about 5 years into the FEDS' evolution, we began noticing—and grew concerned about—how our participants were disproportionately female (60%–70%). This was happening at the same time that the major funders of health disparities scholarship were making calls to better engage minority men in health education, outreach, interventions, and programming. We brought this challenge and opportunity to our leadership group and other FEDS participants. What followed was the creation of the (simply called) Men's Group. In a similar manner to the FEDS, it is co-led by community members and professionals. But it differs in not following a set schedule in a single location and by its outdoor activities (vs. the FEDS' mostly indoor programming that has an educational feel). The Men's Group aims to reclaim the valued roles of men in American Indian families, alongside health-related pursuits that reflect Native cultures. Primarily affiliated with a local American Indian Family Center, activities include community gatherings with sacred offerings, smudging, prayer, drumming, singing, dancing, talking circles, and public conversations and sharing between men about a host of topics relevant to historical trauma and colonization, living in contemporary Western culture, coping with stressors such as poverty and unemployment, and collectively "taking back" valued traditional practices that have been lost along the way. The Men's Group has repaired and built sweat lodges together. They grow wild rice together (including all the activities involved, such as picking, collecting, cutting wood for roasting, and preparing). They harvest maple syrup (sugar-bushing). They organize fishing groups (including ice fishing in the winter) and have formed softball and basketball teams, playing in tournaments during the summertime. These activities involve collective support for healthy living, infused by a strong sense of spirituality (connecting the men's efforts with their Creator, Ancestors, and people) and dignity (as valued leaders, role models, and sources of support for youth and other men).

Second, it was also becoming clear to us in the FEDS that the majority of our participants were adults. Older parents and their adult children were actively engaged in the program, but parents of minor children pointed out that their youngsters did not find the FEDS particularly fun because the education, discussions, and activities within it were a better fit for "old people." This was troubling because diabetes among American Indian children is strikingly common and because healthy behaviors are best begun early in life.

We brought this challenge to our leadership group and other FEDS participants. What followed was the creation of our community's Youth Education, co-led by community members (adult and youth) and professionals. Like the Men's Group, it does not follow a set schedule in a single location, and it emphasizes its outdoor activities. Primarily affiliated with our local community's Ain Dah Yung Center and Saint Paul Public Schools American Indian Education Program, it integrates culturally based notions of walking in balance with empirically supported knowledge about young people's health and disease management. Youth participate in traditional recreation and games, construct and maintain a medicine garden, run education booths at local powwows, and regularly take part in Native dance. They also work hard to bring back new learnings and activities to their homes through discussions with parents, siblings, cousins, and other family members.

Beyond the unique features that make each of these interventions unique and innovative, all of our activities—including the FEDS, Men's Group, and Youth Education—are designed to offer overlaps in participation. From our Men's Group, many of the men's wives/partners and relatives (and some of the men, themselves) participate in the FEDS, and many of their children participate in our youth interventions. From our Youth Education, children are encouraged to bring what they learn back into their families, and many of the children's parents go on to participate in our Men's Group and FEDS program. As all members in all of these groups work to walk in balance, they do so in a way that creates a whole that is greater than the sum of its parts.

3 STUDENTS AGAINST NICOTINE AND TOBACCO ADDICTION

The project described in this chapter is a health promotion initiative that was cocreated through the efforts of medical and mental health professionals with students, educators, and administrators at the Hubert H. Humphrey Job Corps Center in Saint Paul, Minnesota. Guided by the citizen health care model, the Students Against Nicotine and Tobacco Addiction (SANTA) project involved multiple interventions to reduce the stress and boredom that students think smoking will alleviate, alongside changes to the Job Corps campus environment, on-site rules and policies, and its formal smoking cessation and peer support resources.

Several publications during the early years of SANTA's creation and evaluation phases tell the full story of this initiative (Mendenhall et al., 2010, 2011; Mendenhall, Harper, et al., 2014; Mendenhall, Whipple, et al., 2008). What follows below is an abbreviated version of these narratives, with special attention to how pairing young adults' wisdom, lived experience, and energy with conventional health programming changed long-standing and

https://doi.org/10.1037/0000378-004
Becoming a Citizen Therapist: Integrating Community Problem-Solving Into Your Work as a Healer, by W. J. Doherty and T. J. Mendenhall

heretofore unsuccessful efforts to improve health behaviors among students in the Job Corps community, many of whom are at high risk for high school dropout, unemployment, or underemployment (National Job Corps Association, 2023).

ORIGINS OF THE SANTA PROJECT

The Job Corps was established by the U.S. Department of Labor in the 1960s to provide high-quality academic and trade-skills training in a safe living environment for at-risk youth and young adults (ages 15–24 years). The on-site health and wellness centers, counseling centers, and center standards and incentives offices at Job Corps centers across the nation work to support students in these pursuits through job shadowing and field placements that offer hands-on learning in a wide range of professions (e.g., facilities maintenance, machining, electrical, plumbing, culinary arts). In the early 2000s, internal focus groups and survey data at the Minnesota-based Job Corps revealed that more than 40% of its students smoked cigarettes, with significant increases in tobacco use after arriving on campus. Nearly 70% of these students reported unsuccessful efforts in smoking cessation (Haas, 2005).

All of this was very concerning, of course, but not just for the obvious health dangers of smoking. Job Corps administrators were worried because they knew that applicants for new positions were less competitive if they arrived at interviews smelling like smoke (Dusheck, 2016; Michalek et al., 2020; Prochaska et al., 2016). Put simply, potential employers prefer employees who they presume will cost them less in future health care troubles and miss less work due to sick days. Job Corps teachers were worried because students who smoked were more frequently late for class after running back and forth from the designated on-campus smoking area during breaks. They also perceived these students to be less engaged in and on pace with what they were teaching, which could also affect their future employability. Job Corps health providers were worried for all of the health implications that smoking brings with it. Job Corps students (200–250 at any given time, 90% of whom reside in on-campus dormitories) were worried about their own or their friends' health, alongside their future employability. For different and overlapping reasons, everyone recognized this problem as one that they shared in common. And because years of conventional antismoking information campaigns, nicotine replacement therapies, and formal quit plans had proven unsuccessful at Job Corps, receptivity to new ideas was high.

As I (Tai) began to meet with Job Corps' administration, teachers, and health providers, I introduced the citizen health care approach as a novel way to address students' smoking. Recognizing that the voices missing from this conversation were those of Job Corps students, I encouraged teachers and health providers to think about who to invite. They then asked a number of students who were well-liked and highly trusted among their peers to join a planning group consisting of 16 students (10 who did not smoke and six who did), four faculty members, two health providers, and two University of Minnesota faculty (I and a close physician colleague).

PROGRAM CONTENT AND PROCESSES

Our first several meetings involved participants getting to know and gain trust with one another. No group at Job Corps had ever included such a diversity of stakeholders, nor had students ever collaborated with administrators or faculty in a flattened hierarchy and collaborative manner. United in concerns about smoking, the first products of their work evolved through the creation of a name (Students Against Nicotine and Tobacco Addiction) and shared purpose: "Our mission is to improve the health and well-being of students at Job Corps through smoking cessation, education, stress reduction, and support."

Over the next year, SANTA leadership group participants (all of them) cocreated a recurring series of surveys and assessments to inform questions about (a) why students smoke, (b) what stresses students the most (because stress is so often paired with smoking), (c) which SANTA interventions students might engage with the most, and (d) readiness to change (paired with actual change) related to smoking. They also developed strategies for program sustainability so that SANTA could live on after sequential cohorts of student and professional members left Job Corps via graduation or retirement.

In response to campus-wide surveys confirming that students primarily smoked as a means to manage stress (or combat boredom), it became clear why previous interventions that targeted smoking behaviors only, without addressing the underlying motivations to smoke, had not been effective. Student members then worked to create and lead new activities that targeted stress (or boredom) reduction as a means to circumvent smoking, with cessation as a beneficial "side effect." Dancing, rap contests, yoga, basketball, volleyball, running, and other physically active activities and groups began to gain in popularity as after-class and weekend options for students. Other, less physically active activities and groups also took form, including those aligned with theater or drama, chess, art, and a book club. Students created posters to advertise these activities and posted them in dormitories and other shared spaces. Job Corps administrators supported these efforts through accommodation of space, announcing and describing them in campus assembles, and contributing other resources and supplies. Anecdotally (at first) and formally (later), students confirmed that participating in these activities contributed to reductions in stress, boredom, and smoking.

As SANTA's leaders queried multiple generations of the student body (as old students graduated and new students came to campus) about their stress, they found the most commonly cited sources were financial problems, job searching, feeling homesick, family conflict, and personal problems (e.g., health worries, relationship troubles). In response to this knowledge, they created a new campus newsletter called the *SANTA Report* to share information and strategies to allay these struggles. This resource was kept current and distributed to all students (individually in their mailboxes and collectively on large posters strategically placed in busy parts of campus) once per month. SANTA students and professionals also began to host and present at education forums to teach and talk about how to strategically manage finances, seek employment, and navigate interpersonal conflict and where to seek help in safe and confidential ways. We created ways for students to connect with other students in 1:1 formats for peer support and added group meetings to standardized support formats for smoking cessation. At the same time, the leadership group took the bold step, with the support of administrators, of moving the campus-designated smoking area to a less desirable location on the very edge of campus and requiring that staff who wished to smoke do so in their cars (outside of students' view). SANTA also designed SANTA t-shirts and buttons and received permission for these to be worn instead of otherwise required school uniforms. This served to further increase SANTA's visibility on campus. Anecdotally (at first) and formally (later), students confirmed that these and related program efforts contributed to reductions in stress, boredom, and smoking.

To advance SANTA's appeal and sustainability with an ever-changing student body, the group continued to administer campus-wide surveys to inform which activities to maintain versus discontinue (in accord with what students perceived as most engaging). Evaluations of health behaviors continued to track smoking, paired with assessments regarding which activities were most facilitative of health behavior change and readiness to change.

SANTA'S UNCONVENTIONAL STRATEGIES

Most health messaging about cigarettes has used scare or shaming tactics in hopes of dissuading people from using tobacco products. Given numerous messages with large print (in the United States) on packaging, billboards, buses, and public benches that warn against cancer and miscarriages and graphic pictures of diseased tissue and rotting teeth (in other countries), it is doubtful that smokers are unaware of these risks. However, research also shows that such messaging is generally not effective at promoting healthy behavior change (Brookes & Harvey, 2015; Guttman & Salmon, 2004).

This knowledge, from both formal scholarship and lay wisdom, was discussed at length during the early phases of SANTA's efforts. We did not want what we were doing to be an on-campus campaign by nonsmokers to change the behaviors of smokers because nonsmokers "knew best" or were otherwise superior by way of narratives such as "If you smoke, you smell bad," "You're wasting money," or "Why are you doing something that you know is so unhealthy?" Furthermore, we knew that endeavors to tap the lived experience and wisdom of students (heretofore missing from Job Corps' efforts to reduce on-campus smoking) needed to include the voices of both nonsmokers and smokers. And although several members of the leadership team were resistant to the idea at first, they quickly agreed with the notion that the only way to authentically understand the experience(s) of an addiction was to have personal experience with one.

And so, as already mentioned, when Job Corps faculty and staff brainstormed about who to invite from the student body, they knew they had to invite smokers. This proved to be helpful in several ways initially and over the long haul. Early conversations in SANTA engaged smokers and nonsmokers through discourse that resisted conventional us-versus-them thinking. Surveys designed to engage everyone on campus about why some students smoke and others do not, what drives smoking, and ways to target stress and boredom reflected the efforts of everyone involved. The optics of SANTA's smoking and nonsmoking members working together to administer surveys, followed by the collaborative nature of interventions it created, showed how we were all invested in everyone's health.

As a project born out of citizen health care, SANTA was not, therefore, a conventional smoking cessation program, which is typically a clinical service (a) led by nonsmoking expert providers engaged with smoking patients, (b) informed by principles of motivational interviewing and readiness to change, (c) oriented toward an official quit date, and (d) followed up with a variety of supportive efforts to maintain beneficent change. Indeed, Job Corps providers were quick to say early on that conventional top-down approaches were not working.

Instead, SANTA was a community-owned and -operated program that engaged the contributions of providers and students in partnership with each other. It targeted stress and boredom more than it targeted smoking. It did this because Job Corps students told us that stress and boredom are the primary problems and impetuses of said smoking. As SANTA's constellation of programming advanced in response to this call, students' stress and boredom went down (see next section), and so did smoking.

IMPACT AND FOLLOW-UP

SANTA participants were interested in assessing the impact of their efforts from the very beginning, in large part because of a shared sense of urgency to do something vis-à-vis (a) historically ineffective efforts to reduce on-campus smoking by administrators and other Job Corps staff and (b) an often-expressed despondence by students about how difficult it is to quit. The activities that SANTA created to reduce stress and boredom, paired with the changes that it promoted in Job Corps' physical environment and smoking-related policies, carried strong face validity and reason for hope. But we needed formal data that went beyond anecdotal or individual accounts about how the program was helpful. We needed data regarding the overall prevalence of smoking at Job Corps and to track whether it was going down because of SANTA's endeavors.

Collecting these data was difficult, however, because of the revolving-door nature of any sample we could engage at any one time. New students were always enrolling at Job Corps and thus had not been exposed to SANTA for very long, and more senior students were always graduating after a year or more of exposure. As a consequence, assessments of the whole student body never evidenced significant change. However, as our team tracked unique cohorts of students, we found that smoking initially increased (presumably because of stressors previously mentioned and adjusting to a new environment) and then consistently decreased for the duration of their stay at Job Corps. More sophisticated analyses later on found that positive shifts in readiness to change were happening for students who had not yet reported actual behavioral changes in smoking. We found, too, that SANTA's physical activities (such as volleyball and running) were the most popular but that its nonphysical activities (art, theater, seminars) were the most influential in promoting positive outcomes. SANTA's other efforts (e.g., changes to the physical environment) were also significantly associated with the cohort-by-cohort outcomes that we sought. For a detailed description of these evaluations, see Mendenhall, Harper, et al. (2014).

PROJECT END AND INTEGRATION OF ACTIVITIES

SANTA was an innovative and welcome initiative at the Minnesota-based Job Corps. Over time, it was recognized as the longest lasting student-engaged program on campus. No doubt this was due to members' deep investment to sustain the program long after their own graduation, retirement, and/or change in workplace role, position, or location. Multiple generations of students, key professionals, teachers, and administrators were involved in the program over the years. Program leaders were successful in securing large grants to formally evaluate its efforts, but later the work was carried on without programmatic funding because its members believed in SANTA's mission.

In the late 2010s (2017–2019), after navigating multiple changes in Job Corps' administrative ownership and restructuring, SANTA as a formal project began to sunset. Remaining, however, was the energy that we have consistently found with citizen health care initiatives that include teenagers (Mendenhall & Doherty, 2007a; Mendenhall et al., 2015). Campus-wide efforts and attention to programming that is not wholly academic endure. This is important because students generally reside on campus. If there is nothing to do besides go to classes or participate in job-training activities, then the boredom and stress of dormitory living and otherwise limited mobility can put students at increased risk for a variety of unhealthy trajectories. But the buffet of physical and nonphysical activities that Job Corps offers its students lives on, and these undoubtedly benefit them across both mental and physical well-being. Less stress and less boredom translate into less smoking and healthier living.

4

THE COMO CLINIC HEALTH CLUB

Activating Citizen Patient Leaders

Our first citizen health care projects, described in Chapters 2 and 3, focused on specific health issues such as diabetes and cigarette smoking. The project described in this chapter came from an interest in whether citizen health care could engage patients with a variety of health challenges. In other words, could people cocreate a health promotion initiative when their direct experience with a specific illness or health challenge was not the focus?

As we formulated this interest in 2009, we were aware of the development of health care homes, a promising innovation in the organization of primary care in the United States. (It's also called the *patient-centered medical home.*) The federal Agency for Healthcare Research and Quality (2012) defined the health care home as a delivery mode involving five characteristics: comprehensive, patient-centered, coordinated, accessible, and high quality. In its ideal form, a wide range of clinicians work in collaborative teams with patients and families to improve health outcomes and quality of life for people living with chronic health conditions and disabilities.

An acknowledged weak area in health care homes is the engagement of patients individually in their own health care and communities more generally (Nutting et al., 2011; Reibling, 2016). Health care homes have focused

https://doi.org/10.1037/0000378-005
Becoming a Citizen Therapist: Integrating Community Problem-Solving Into Your Work as a Healer, by W. J. Doherty and T. J. Mendenhall

on building collaborative provider systems, not on actively engaging patients in their own health care. This is no small gap because there is general consensus that unless patients and families become more responsible for their own health promotion and health care, the economics of health care will become unsustainable (Graffigna, 2017).

To address this key pressure point in the health care system, I (Bill) began working with HealthPartners' Como Clinic, a large primary care clinic, to create a strong patient engagement arm of their health care home, a project that eventually was named the Como Clinic Health Club. When this project began, Tai and I were 10 years into citizen therapist work and able to bring a well-defined, step-by-step approach to the launching phase. This chapter focuses on the startup phase to demonstrate how a citizen therapist project using our model can be put on the ground. We then give an overview of specific activities of the Como Clinic Health Club.

ORIGIN OF THE PROJECT

The idea of engaging a primary care clinic that was developing a health care home came from brainstorming conversations I (Bill) had with several local health care innovators. Perhaps patients could organize around a clinic they shared in common even if they did not share the same health care challenges. My colleagues steered me to physician Steve Radosevich, a general internist and medical director of a 25,000-patient clinic that was part of HealthPartners, which is a large nonprofit health care system in Minnesota. Steve had a background as an innovator and was well-connected in the HealthPartners system.

I clearly recall my first conversations with Steve. I told him I had just come from a meeting with the principal and lead teacher in a public elementary school with a large population of African immigrant students. I told Steve that when I asked if they could recommend a dozen parent leaders in the school who might be interested in a project, the principal and teacher immediately said, "No problem." There were many parents already volunteering in the school and providing leadership in the parent–teacher association. With a smile indicating I knew I was asking the impossible from Steve as the medical director, I added, "I imagine that if I asked you to come up with a dozen *patient leaders,* you'd be stumped." He smiled back and shook his head in agreement. I went on: "The term *patient leader* is nearly an oxymoron in health care. Patients come as individuals or families for their own care; there are no opportunities for them to participate in the mission of the clinic."

The central idea of this new project, I said, was to see if a primary care clinic could be like a small town where townspeople have a role in promoting the well-being of the community irrespective of their personal health situations. This would mean creating a citizen health care team of patients working with medical professionals to cocreate a project. I made a distinction between three kinds of citizen involvement:

- input: offering advice to professionals who are creating a new program (this is done sometimes by patient advisory boards),

- feedback: patients evaluating the services already provided (this is done routinely now in health care), and

- cocreation: patients and professionals developing a new project together with shared leadership (this is the focus of citizen health care).

Steve readily took to the cocreation idea, noting that Como Clinic in Saint Paul was one of the first prepaid health maintenance organization (HMO) clinics in the nation back in the 1950s and had even had a patient governing board in those days. Steve had elderly patients in his own practice who were leaders in those early days. Como Clinic would be an ideal place to reflect professionals as authority figures. Numbers are important too: The lay citizen members of the leadership group should outnumber the professionals by at least 3:1; otherwise, the sheer proportion of professionals is apt to inhibit the sense of co-ownership of the project by patient members.

The next step was to decide how to recruit the patient members. The small staff group and I met twice to generate criteria for which patients to invite and to decide on a recruitment method. The criteria were as follows:

- members of the clinic (bonus if also a parent or caregiver of a clinic member)
- a variety of age groups
- interested in own health and invested in this clinic community
- a variety of lengths of contact with the clinic
- would appear to be comfortable in a group process
- ethnic diversity
- gender balance
- some parents of children in the clinic

Several of these criteria were straightforward and easy to determine, while others depended on the intuition of the clinician seeing the patient. An example of intuition is something like this: During an annual physical the patient offers thoughts or asks questions about how the overall clinic is doing or brings up public health issues in addition to their own personal health. In other words, the patient shows an interest in health care. Another example would be whether the clinician could picture the patient as contributing constructively to a group process. The three professional members of the group developed their own invitation lists of patients and invited a couple of other like-minded providers to develop theirs as well.

Tai and I had learned from other projects that people are gratified to be nominated by their clinician for a leadership role. (Most contacts from one's provider are about test results or other personal medical information.) The staff group and I composed a letter that would come from the clinician that would emphasize the patient's potential to contribute to an exciting new project in the clinic and be personally signed. The letter was followed by a call from one of three professionals on the planning team expressing hope that the patient would consider participating. Here is the text of the letter:

Dear _____:

I am writing to see if you would like to be part of a new project at Como Clinic. The project will bring together providers and patient leaders to create a new way for patients and families to be more deeply involved in their own health care and that of the Como Clinic community. The project would be the first of its kind, as far as we know.

I am nominating you for the ongoing planning group for this project because I see you as interested in health care and having the personal qualities the planning group can use. An informational meeting is scheduled for Wednesday, April 14 at 7 p.m. to fill in the details of what is involved in the project. One of the providers on the planning group will call you soon to see if you are interested in attending.

I see this collaborative project as an important opportunity to make a difference for our health community, and I hope you will consider being part of it. Of course I will understand if you cannot put anything else on your plate right now.

Sincerely,

[Provider signature]

Note that this letter invites people to an informational meeting that would serve as a launch event for the project. An informational meeting gives people the spirit of the project along with an understanding of what the commitment would be. Exhibit 4.1 shows the plan for the meeting at Como Clinic. The design involved a lot of participant engagement in the first part, with people introducing themselves, saying which provider invited them, how long they have been at the clinic, and why they accepted the invitation to come to this meeting. Then there was a brief presentation of the challenge in health care to achieve deep engagement of patients, followed by discussion and reaction to these ideas. Then I described the citizen health care model as an alternative to the traditional way to think about provider–consumer health care,

EXHIBIT 4.1. Plan for the Launch Event

COMO CITIZEN PATIENT PROJECT ORIENTATION MEETING
April 14, 2010, 7-9 p.m.

1. Welcome and orientation to the meeting

   Goals of this meeting

   - To inform patient leaders about a new Citizen Health Project at Como. The project will develop new ways for patients at Como to become more deeply involved in their own health care and that of the clinic community.
   - To recruit patient members for a Citizen Health Care Action Group that will plan and implement the project over the next year

2. Introductions

   - Name and role: patient (and who nominated you), staff, process leader, observer
   - How long have you been connected to Como Clinic?

3. Why everyone is here

   - Patients first: Why did you accept the invitation to come to this meeting?
   - Professionals: What's your own interest in this project?

4. The pressure point in the health care system

   - Health care reform is in the air, but it's been mostly insurance- and provider-oriented thus far. Nearly everyone agrees that we won't have high-quality, affordable health care unless patients take more responsibility for their own health. Otherwise, health care reform will promise what the system can't deliver.
   - For years we have emphasized the importance of patient engagement, patient self-responsibility, or patient self-management, but this work stays mainly at the individual level—patients and their own doctor in the exam room. We have not yet learned how to tap the *collective energies* of patients who are citizens of health care for themselves and their communities.
   - Health care improvement initiatives in medical settings are designed by professionals and delivered to patients. Seldom are patients invited to gather as coproducers of initiatives to address problems in the health care community.

   Question: What reactions and reflections do you have to this statement of the problem or pressure point in health care?

5. Explanation of the citizen health care model (handout)

6. Idea of the citizen patient project (handout)

   - How does this approach to the project sound to you?
   - Do you think it could benefit the health of individuals and the community?
   - Questions about what is involved for those who participate

7. Invitation to join the project

   - The first Citizen Health Care Action Group meeting will be Wednesday, April 28, 7:00-8:30 p.m. in Conference Room B.
   - Sign-up sheets handed out

8. How do you feel about what we've done here tonight?

followed by an explanation of the new citizen patient project and questions from the group. At the end there was an opportunity to sign up for the project and commit to attending the first working meeting 2 weeks hence. We've learned to invite people to a specific time for the beginning of the leadership group (usually the same day of the week and time of the launch event) rather than try to mesh everyone's schedules. Once the group is launched, members can modify the meeting schedule.

About 30 patients attended the informational launch event, of whom a surprising number (20) signed up for the project and attended the first working group meeting. (Over the next 18 months, normal attrition reduced the group to a more manageable size of 12–15.) The launch event experience was powerful for patient participants and the professional group who planned it. Patients were highly enthusiastic about being part of an innovation in health care. They seemed eager to cocreate a project in partnership with the three clinic staff members who participated. (I introduced myself as the process leader.) Having said that, we did not end up with the diversity we had hoped for. The few parents of young children who attended the launch event did not commit to the project because of other demands on their time. Only one patient who was a person of color attended the launch event (an African immigrant woman), and she did sign on to the project. (The clinic population is largely White.) Most of the patients who entered the project were late-career or early-retirement individuals who had time to give back to the clinic community. Despite efforts to diversify the leadership group over the next decade, the demographics remained largely the same, something that clearly is a limitation of the project.

THE EARLY PROCESS OF COCREATING A PROJECT

Consistent with the citizen health care model, the project leadership group took time to go deep over the ensuing months before deciding on its first action steps. We focused on three core questions, summarized below. (Exhibit 4.2 contains the full summary of what the group generated from the questions.) As process leader I wrote down what the group developed and discussed, clarified, and revised over several meetings.

- Even in a health care system (like Como Clinic) that provides good access and quality professional care, what are the main challenges we face in staying healthy and managing illness? Responses were categorized into personal challenges, cultural challenges, and challenges in dealing with even a good, accessible health care system.

EXHIBIT 4.2. Analysis of Limitations of Current Health Care and How Patients Can Engage

What Health Care Professionals Traditionally Do

- Provide information over and over
- Encourage, persuade patients to take better care of themselves
- Offer public education campaigns and public service announcements
- Support government laws (on smoking, seat belts, helmet use, others)
- Encourage primary care providers to spend time on prevention and educate patients
- Refer to programs such as Alcoholics Anonymous, WeightWatchers, YMCA
- Recently, encourage use of the internet, Web 2.0
- Refer to some team-based and home-based services to help people live with chronic illness

Limitations and Barriers in the Traditional Approach

Provider Side

- Having to see a lot of patients quickly
- Rapidly changing knowledge base
- Easier to address immediate needs, harder to address broader ones
- Traditional emphasis on diagnosis and disease
- Focus on technical interventions: measure, test, medicate, or do surgery
- Evidence-based medicine can lead to missing the individuality of patients
- Routines of health care can make it predictable but miss the patient
- Lack of coordinated teams who can share the work of health promotion
- Traditionally, not seeing mental health as key in health promotion
- Clinicians don't have a variety of tools in health promotion
- Stereotypes and biases about groups of patients
- Some patients want traditional, provider-driven care
- Some patients are not trustworthy in what they report to providers
- Clinicians can't be all things to all people
- It's hard to think outside the box of traditional models of working with patients

Patient Side

- A lot of information coming at patients, from many sources
- So much talking, like raindrops in a bucket
- Patients don't remember what providers say
- Health care is often "done to" the patient
- Patients are not empowered individually or collectively
- Individual differences among patients are often not attended to; instead, one size fits all
- Cultural norms affecting health are not brought up and dealt with
- Many patients are used to being "acted upon" (reflecting cultural norms)
- Providers and insurance designed systems that patients have to access rather than belong to

(continues)

EXHIBIT 4.2. Analysis of Limitations of Current Health Care and How Patients Can Engage (*Continued*)

- Health care without caring does not inspire patients to change
- Some patients don't have access to resources their providers encourage (such as fresh food and the internet)
- Patient biases and stereotypes about providers and what they do
- Patients not trusting providers and the care system in the face of conflicting information and past experiences
- Patient experience of fragmented health care
- Messages of popular culture that we pass on to one another

How We Manage Our Health Together

Health refers to staying healthy and handling illness well.

- Family pressures to take care of ourselves
- Doing healthy things with one another, such as walking together
- Family meals
- Healthy cooking at home
- Providing emotional support, listening
- Motivating each other
- Paying attention to how people in our lives are looking and acting
- Sharing knowledge and treatment ideas, including home remedies and self-education ideas
- Telling stories, sharing experiences about health challenges
- Finding and connecting with someone else with the same problem
- Online connecting with people with similar challenges
- Providing direct care
- Advocating for each other
- Offering support through prayer lines, CaringBridge
- Donating blood
- Community programs such as health fairs and blood drives that have active involvement of community members
- Helping others get to medical appointments
- Helping people to understand their medical bills

- In our traditional way of doing health care, how do we try to help people overcome the personal and cultural challenges to staying healthy and managing illness well? A follow-up question: What are the barriers and limitations to doing this traditional approach? Responses were categorized into provider barriers (What keeps them from doing traditional approaches to health promotion well?) and patient barriers (What keeps them from making good use of traditional approaches?).

- Aside from the provider system, how do we manage our health (staying healthy and handling illness well) in our families and communities? This question addressed the informal, family and community part of health care that was the focus of our project. Ways to get into the question included asking (a) Whose health and health challenges do I know about in my social world of family, friends, neighbors, coworkers, faith community members, and so on and (b) How am I part of their efforts to stay healthy and manage illness well, and how are they part of mine?

The initial name for the project was the Active Member Project, reflecting an emphasis on active engagement and the use of the term *member* by Health-Partners as a cooperative, nonprofit health care organization with a member-elected board. Later the leadership group renamed the project the Como Clinic Health Club, which emphasizes the informal nature of the project—a club rather than a project. The original mission statement stuck: "To engage patients of all ages as active agents of their own health and well-being, and as citizens of the Como Clinic community." We recite this mission statement at the outset of each meeting, along with what we call our central premise: "The greatest untapped resource for improving health and health care is the knowledge, wisdom, and energy of individuals, families, and communities who face challenging health issues in their everyday lives."

A key ingredient in any citizen health care project is discerning which potential action steps are consistent with the model. This has to occur before people begin to generate action ideas, lest proposals come forward that have to be rejected because they fit traditional top-down, provider–consumer approaches and not a horizontal, patient-led model. So, before the group generated action steps, we agreed on the criteria we would use for deciding whether an action idea was consistent with the model we were using. To repeat, this is important as a way to prevent lapsing back into traditional provider–consumer approaches. The six criteria are that the activity

- reflects the mission of engaging patients as active agents of their own health and well-being and as citizens of the clinic community,
- has a way to tap the knowledge and experience of the people participating— not just a class with a question-and-answer component,
- builds connections among clinic members,
- taps the leadership of club members,
- is accessible to and inclusive of people from diverse populations (age, racial–ethnic background, income level), and
- is feasible without substantial new resources.

Consulting these criteria saved the group a number of times from creating activities that would compromise our framework, such as inviting a medical specialist to present slides on a health issue and then take questions. Instead, the group developed processes to ensure group interaction and mutual teaching and learning in every club activity. We decided that a great way to make the new project visible in the clinic community was to sponsor a cookout lunch with a meet-and-greet in the clinic parking lot. It was billed as a healthy grilling event for staff and patients from 11 a.m. to 1:30 p.m., with recipes handed out for the food and opportunities for patients and staff to sign up for our newsletter and to learn about upcoming events.

HEALTH CLUB ACTIVITIES

For the first few years the Como Clinic Health Club held monthly or bimonthly events but struggled to get visibility in the clinic because we had only limited staff support from a clinic secretary for advertising and coordinating the logistics for events. After HealthPartners leaders came to realize that the club was doing something valuable and innovative, we were able to gain an important resource: a professional staff member (Jennette Turner, a health coach by training) who could devote 2 days per week to coordinating the logistics of the health club: the website, the email list, the monthly newsletter, room sign-up, and helping to recruit new patient leaders. At that point, which was Year 3 of the project, the health club really took off, engaging hundreds of patients per year. Following is a partial list of activities:

- TED Talk group conversations on a variety of topics (e.g., mindfulness, caregiving, disease prevention, end-of-life issues). (The group watched a TED Talk chosen by the leadership team and then had structured group conversations about the topics.)

- cooking classes that engaged patients in preparing meals

- end-of-life workshops led by a patient leader with a strong personal interest in the topic

- yoga classes taught by a clinic patient

- a clinic garden planned, planted, tended, and harvested by patients and clinic staff members

- a walking club

- annual healthy grilling event: about 250 healthy meals served to patients and staff

- poetry and health group led by a staff physician with a passion for poetry
- interactive workshops on "political stress" and how to talk with loved ones across the political chasm
- biking outings and workshops
- a children's bookshelf in the pediatric waiting room
- workshops on a variety of topics including racial equity and health, gun issues and health, and climate change and health

These activities emerged from the monthly leadership team meetings on the basis of group interest, fit with the citizen health care model, and whether a citizen patient leader was willing to champion the activity. The patient leadership turned over several times over the 12 years of the project, with new leaders invited from among Como patients who attended events and showed an interest in continuing the work of the project. Three original members remain from the group who launched the project. Around Year 5, HealthPartners commissioned an evaluation of the Como Clinic Health Club. (Details follow.)

In 2020 HealthPartners leaders decided that the model was promising enough to disseminate to other clinics. Coordinator Jennette Turner and I met with professional leaders at two other clinics in the HealthPartners system to begin the same launching process we used at Como: orienting professionals, recruiting patient leaders, and a launch event. One of those health clubs gained traction right away, and the other struggled to retain enough patient leaders in the core team. One difference seemed to be that the successful clinic, like Como, was neighborhood- and community-based primary care whereas the other was a multispecialty clinic that drew patients from a wide geographical region.

Evaluation of the project took two forms: (a) documentation of the process of implementation and patient uptake of the activities and (b) a survey of clinic patients in 2017 to determine how visible the health club had become and the level of participation and satisfaction of those who participated in the activities. For the first kind of evaluation, I developed detailed notes of the process we used (as reflected in this chapter). For the second kind, the survey indicated that about 25% of the 25,000 patients in the clinic were aware of the health club, and of that total about 15% had participated in its activities. Those who participated rated the activities highly for promoting their health. The visibility finding demonstrated a problem that has still never been resolved, namely, that we are not allowed access to the whole patient population through email or other electronic means. The rationale for the policy is that clinic communications with patients should be confined to the patient's own medical situations. It's clear that we had not yet influenced the overall patient engagement model of HealthPartners.

THE COVID PANDEMIC SHUTDOWN AND THE END OF THE PROJECT

The pandemic that began in 2020 was a blow to the health club project. HealthPartners shut down the project and laid off Jennette. The Como Club and the other two health clubs went into hibernation for about 10 months and were nearly terminated by the HealthPartners division that had provided the staff support. Steve Radosevich stepped down as clinic director, and the new director was less interested in the project at a time of great stress for all medical clinics. However, I had connections with the top leader in HealthPartners, who asked the division that had funded the project coordinator to find a way to keep it going with another staff member. We then met for a year via Zoom and held a dozen or so Zoom events. In August 2022 we returned to meeting in person, reduced in numbers because some citizen patient leaders had drifted away but prepared to reboot the project.

After the first draft of this chapter was written, HealthPartners permanently closed down the Como Clinic Health Club and the other two clubs, citing lack of traction in regaining momentum after the pandemic (albeit with much more limited resources) and budgetary priorities. The leadership group met for a last time to debrief about our time together and the ending. A key factor in the ending of the project was the transition at the HealthPartners leadership level from our initial key supporters to another leadership cohort who inherited the project and never owned it as something they fully embraced. Even though most of the work was done by patients, the health club was nevertheless a cost center (most via a part-time coordinator) and not a revenue center for the organization. With champions gone at the clinic and management/leadership levels, the project was vulnerable to cutbacks happening all over the system.

Perhaps a 12-year ride in a big health care system with turnover of middle managers and senior leaders was as much as could be expected. Having said that, a lesson is that we could have lobbied those managers and leaders more intentionally to get them behind the project. We had institutional champions at the outset, but when they departed, we did not work hard enough to gain new champions among their replacements. The final debrief with the health club leadership group was both sad and heartwarming as we reflected on a sense of satisfaction for contributions to the clinic community, personal connections, and a sense of becoming leaders for promoting health. Mary Griffith, one of the founding members, sent these words to me about her experience:

> I've been with the Como Health Club since its inception. I truly believe that the communities we are in (schools, jobs, neighborhoods, churches, etc.) can shape and change our lives, so it made sense to me to have a community that supports good health and health care. As we explored the initial idea, I was impressed by the methodical and efficient process that clarified exactly what we were trying to do. I'm willing to commit my time to the leadership group because I see the same commitment in members with differing strengths and interests. I only have to put my efforts toward projects I'm really excited about, which keeps me from getting burned out. At the same time, participating in so many of our projects has made me healthier and more knowledgeable about the health care available to me.
>
> I am constantly surprised by what we achieved together. We've come up with very creative and useful programs that have achievable goals. The response we get from participants fuels my enthusiasm for this health club. Communities create support; it's hard to be motivated in isolation. Every event and effort we make reaches more than the participants. Every person who reads our newsletter, eats at our grilling event, takes a book from the children's free book cart, or picks the basil in our garden gets the message "We care about you and your health. We care about each other."

Activated citizens tend to keep going even when formal projects close down. The club's walking group decided to continue, and someone stepped up to manage a Facebook group to help people stay connected. This project was about promoting resilience via patient leadership and mutual support. The resilience continues.

PART **III** FAMILY AND
CULTURAL
CHANGE
PROJECTS

5

PUTTING FAMILY FIRST

Resisting the Pull of Overscheduling Kids

The citizen therapist project described in this chapter is different from our other work in two ways. First, it focused on larger cultural norms affecting middle-class families. In the world of therapy, cultural norms tend to be backgrounded to the presenting concerns of clients (there is no *Diagnostic and Statistical Manual of Mental Disorders* diagnosis for cultural ills), although we may help clients personally resist social norms that may be causing them stress or driving their behavior. Second, professionals involved in community action rarely focus on the concerns of highly resourced individuals and families. In describing the Putting Family First Project, we show how a citizen therapist (Bill) organized parents to name and counter a cultural pathology of middle-class families: overscheduled kids and hyper-competition. This project is described elsewhere in Doherty and Carlson (2002), Doherty (2003), and Anderson and Doherty (2005).

https://doi.org/10.1037/0000378-006
Becoming a Citizen Therapist: Integrating Community Problem-Solving Into Your Work as a Healer, by W. J. Doherty and T. J. Mendenhall

ORIGIN OF PUTTING FAMILY FIRST

Recall that in the introduction to this book we emphasized how parents were experiencing family life as a rat race of activities they felt they had limited power to avoid. This was documented by studies and surveys showing rapid changes toward being highly scheduled that were limiting family time and unstructured time for children (Anderson & Doherty, 2005; S. L. Brown et al., 2011). I (Bill) gave a presentation on the issue in 1998 and decided, along with a community leader, to do a follow-up presentation and a town hall meeting in April 1999. The events were extensively advertised; a large crowd came for the presentation, and a sizable subgroup stayed for the town hall. There was a consensus that the problem of declining family time was a community problem, not just an individual family problem. One (unnamed) participant suggested an idea that became the basis for an important project the next year: our own version of the Good Housekeeping Seal of Approval for organizations that do a good job of supporting family time. At the end of the high-energy town hall meeting, the community leader and I invited parents to sign up for a community action team to provide leadership for a grassroots movement to make family life a higher priority in this community.

A group of about 15 parents met monthly throughout the next year, and I facilitated. We gave a name to the initiative (Putting Family First), went through the process of generating vision and mission statements, and described a desired future for the community. In retrospect, one of our most important tasks was developing a name for the problem—overscheduled kids. This term subsequently entered the American lexicon.

Using a tool of the community organizing tradition, we then did one-to-one stakeholder interviews throughout the community to learn about how others perceive the problem and the ideas and resources these people could bring to the solutions. Members wrote up their interview notes and reported back to the whole group. Some community members joined the Putting Family First leadership group after being interviewed. The interviews convinced the group that we were on the right track in identifying an important community concern.

THE COMMUNITY ACTIONS

We first focused our energies on developing a Putting Family First Seal of Approval for organizations that do a good job of balancing family time with a particular outside activity. After three drafts of the seal, we did more stakeholder interviews, this time concentrating on coaches and other activity leaders whose input and support we needed. We held a special meeting with leaders of several sports leagues to get their input, which was very supportive. These interviews and discussions, which helped us understand both the positive motives and the frustrations of sports leaders, led us to add a section to the seal about the responsibilities of families to the organizations in which they enroll their children.

We were then ready for another public meeting 1 year after the initial public meeting. (This length of time was in keeping with the principle of going deep before taking action. This was held as part of a lecture series on parenting in which I gave a brief presentation based on my new book [Doherty, 2000]). Then I and other members of the Putting Family First leadership group gave an overview of the initiative and the Putting Family First Seal of Approval. The response from the parents attending was intense and enthusiastic.

In the spring and fall of 2000, we developed the application form and procedure for the Putting Family First Seal of Approval. We awarded the first Seal of Approval in January 2001 to the youth football program, after which other community organizations expressed initial interest in the seal. However, the Seal of Approval initiative stalled at that point as other coaches and activity leaders were reluctant to commit to such a public pledge. They said they would follow the spirit of the seal but were concerned about potential downsides from parents who might complain that they were not living up to the pledge.

Realizing we would have to be more proactive in evaluating programs, we then developed a rating guide for dozens of programs based on their published schedules and statements about promoting balance and allowing for family time. We also engaged in conversations with civic leaders and parent–teacher association groups throughout the school district. There was lots of buzz, which was one of our local goals: to start a community-wide conversation.

THE PUBLIC MESSAGING

Even more important than specific community actions was the development of the group's public message. Here is the wording of the three key messages that the group hammered out collectively:

Message #1: The problem. In America today, we are experiencing a problem of overscheduled kids and underconnected families. With the best of intentions for our children's development, we have involved our children in organized activities related to sports, arts, school, and religion. Our communities and society now offer an extraordinary range of choices for our children. In itself, each activity provides the promise of growth and development for our children. And with each activity, we often seek to instill values of achievement, accomplishment, and excellence. Too often, however, the consequence of this competitive and hyperactive parenting has been a loss of family time, a loss of family rituals, and a loss of unstructured time for our children to play, explore, and grow. In fact, every time we say "yes" to a new activity, there is a cost to be paid in terms of family life and family connections.

Message #2: The individual solution. The solution to this problem is to reclaim family time and make family life an honored and celebrated priority. This solution involves two steps. First, we must reclaim family time. Second, we must make good use of that time once we have it back. To reclaim family time, we can set conscious limits on the scheduling of outside activities. And within the home, we can set conscious limits on television, the internet, and other electronic media. We can then consciously and intentionally rebuild family rituals, such as family meals, family vacations, holiday celebrations, family outings, and unstructured family time. Eventually, we can restore a balance between internal bonds and external activities.

Message #3: The community solution. The community must play an essential role in this solution. The Putting Family First initiative is a multi-faceted, grassroots effort to build a community where family life is an honored and celebrated priority. Through the activities, expectations, and policies of its many organizations, the community can be either part of the problem or part of the solution. We are committed to being part of the solution. Our community vision includes the following:

- Schools, faith communities, neighborhoods, and other groups provide families with resources to develop deeper bonds in a fragmenting world.

- Schools, faith communities, neighborhoods, and other groups offer regular intergenerational activities, so that whole families can participate.

- Employers have explicit working policies that honor families' time and energy needs.

- Community activity groups of all kinds have explicit working policies that acknowledge, support, and respect families' decision to make family time a priority.

WHAT WE WANTED TO AVOID IN PUBLIC MESSAGING

The parent leaders were concerned that they not be viewed as superior or judgmental toward other parents in the community. Indeed, some of the parent leaders were receiving comments from other parents justifying why their kids were in, for example, traveling soccer. So, the group developed three norms about what to avoid in our public messages.

- *Creating villains and blaming parents.* The spirit of Putting Family First is that we are all in this problem together and must find a way out together. Coaches are not the enemy, nor is any other group. Parents are doing their best for their children. Individual parents who are overcompetitive are not the problem, because they too are caught up in a broad cultural trend that is spinning out of control. No villains, no scapegoats.

- *Being prescriptive.* Putting Family First is not about telling parents how to manage their time. We suggest no rules such as "one sport at a time." The Putting Family First Seal of Approval does not prohibit practices during the dinner hour. We are calling for reflection about the value of family time and for conscious decisions by families and community organizations about how they intend to foster a balance between family time and outside activities. When parents living highly scheduled lives say, "We like this lifestyle just fine," our response is "Good for you." We aim to influence by attraction, not by prescription. No guilt, no shame.

- *Developing a professionally led program.* Our vision is that families take primary responsibility for Putting Family First, even if a professional such as family therapist guides the process. If you want to hold to this vision, avoid a program approach that focuses on bringing in professionals to conduct classes or workshops. Such educational experiences can be useful as part of a menu of activities but should not be the main course. Putting Family First is not primarily an educational program; it is a grassroots initiative of families to take back family life in a fragmenting world.

These "prohibitions" were particularly helpful when we entered the media attention phase of the work.

MEDIA ATTENTION

Although some local community newspapers had covered Putting Family First public events, a breakthrough occurred when a *New York Times* journalist learned about what was going on in the suburb where the project was located. Here I describe how this happened in some detail to show how citizen therapists can leverage interactions with journalists over standard topics to generate interest in community projects. A veteran *Times* reporter had interviewed me for an article she was writing on marital and couple issues. At the end of the call, I decided to mention "something else I was working on." (The point: When you've done a favor for a journalist by being a good source, they are open to hearing about other possibilities you might offer them.) I mentioned Putting Family First and the problem we were addressing. She immediately lit up, saying that she had observed this phenomenon in her own world and was particularly concerned because she was about to become a mother herself. I emphasized the grassroots nature of the initiative; I was not just a professional with a book on the topic.

The journalist consulted with her editor, who, as fortune would have it, was a mother in the midst of this issue in her own life and community. She greenlighted the journalist for a trip to Minnesota to interview parents, kids, and coaches for several days and write a long and powerful story for the Nation section of the *Times*. The morning the article came out I was awakened early at home by a phone call from a popular local radio show, and my university voice mail was accumulating messages from reporters, local and national. Parents who were interviewed for the article were also getting calls. The leadership group met to talk about how we would respond to the torrent of interest, including a discussion about which of us felt more comfortable with different kinds of interviews. We agreed that one of our members would coordinate media interest, which continued for months and included Oprah, the *Today* show, the major evening news programs, and a great number of talk radio shows. (The Internet was not yet a major source of "going viral" in those days.)

I was glad we had done so much work on our messaging because we were all consistent with how we presented our work, especially in resisting media interest in demonizing "parents who live through their children's accomplishments" and in offering simple prescriptions for what parents should do or not do. The only "enemy" in our messages was a culture that prioritized busyness and competition over family life and balanced childhood, and we invited parents to tune into their own values and avoid just giving into social norms that tell us to love our children mainly by providing competitive activities for them.

My own experience on the *Today* show was a marker in my understanding how a new idea can penetrate the broader society through celebrities. I was waiting off camera for coanchor Katie Couric to interview me. On air at the top of the hour she said, "In this hour, the problem of overscheduled kids." Her colleagues immediately chimed in, "Yes, it's a big problem," and for a minute or so these celebrity figures (including weatherman Al Roker) talked about how they were trying to maintain some balance in their families. Katie Couric said her policy was "one sport at a time" and no more than one evening activity per week.

As I sat waiting for my interview, I told myself, "My job is already done. They've done it for me." But there was more: The *Today* show had followed a family around on its Wednesday afternoon and evening schedule, with three kids and two parents running in different directions and all eating at different times. It was exhausting to watch, although the parents said of their kids, "They like these things. It's not like we are forcing them." Thus we had celebrity testimonials and a powerful video put together with the resources of a TV network. All I had to do was to stay on message—and resist the pulls our group had carefully decided to avoid. I politely resisted Couric's invitation for me to agree that a lot of parents are living through their children. Instead, I said, "I think most parents are trying to do the right thing for their kids in a culture that says more is better." When she asked if whether one evening activity per week was the right policy, I emphasized that every family is different and will have to figure out their own way to have balance. Using my therapist skills, I was able to redirect the interview without seeming to directly contradict her.

Fortunately, that TV segment also featured a video of one of the lead families in Putting Family First, who at one point had been as busy as the other family. It was a striking contrast of kids having unstructured playtime, one organized activity, and, importantly, a family meal. This was an opportunity for the mother to showcase her ability to combine personal experience and our public messages. And of course, she became her own kind of media celebrity as other outlets followed up on the *Today* show segment. Over the next year, the leadership group parents and I were interviewed by print, radio, and TV journalists from around the world.

IMPACT AND FOLLOW-UP

Media messaging was key to our goal of creating a cultural countercurrent to the status quo of parenting. Fortunately, there is a way to indirectly evaluate the impact of Putting Family First on the cultural conversation about kids and families. Google Books Ngram Viewer, which charts the frequency of words across an expansive collection of scanned books written in the English language over the centuries, can be used to track the emergence of novel terms. As mentioned, a key element of Putting Family First was coining a name for a problem that had not been on the cultural radar: overscheduled kids. Entering "overscheduled kids" into Google Books Ngram Viewer shows that it was barely visible in print until Putting Family First began its work in the late 1990s and then made a steep upward climb for a number of years before declining but leveling off at a frequency far above the baseline. In other words, we introduced a term that has now become commonplace in the English language. We named a problem that did not have a name.

Putting Family First was an early harbinger of related movements such as "slow parenting" (Honore, 2009), "free range kids" (Skenaz, 2021), and "human beings versus human doings" (Jarvis, 2016), all of which are attempting to create a countertrend to the still-dominant culture of intense, competitive parenting and other aspects of life. Anecdotally, an adoption social worker with many years of experience interviewing potential adoptive parents told me that she was hearing parents say something new: that they want to provide enrichment activities for a child they would adopt but also want their child to have a balanced life with unstructured time and good family time.

As for Putting Family First as an organization, I moved on to other projects after several years, and the parent leadership started a nonprofit organization and offered resources on balanced childhood and families for another decade before ending its work.

SPIN-OFF PROJECTS

We've learned in our citizen therapist work that sometimes one project spawns another one, as in the case of Partners in Diabetes leading to the Family Education Diabetes Series (FEDS) and the FEDS leading to new projects with men and youth. Putting Family First inspired two additional projects with parents.

Birthdays Without Pressure

The project Birthdays Without Pressure started in nearby Saint Paul as a cultural messaging project on the pressure parents felt about their kids' birthday parties. The initiative emerged from a conversation in a parent education group when a mother complained about how birthday parties were becoming ramped up in work, cost, and expectations for more and better each year. Her comments lit up the group, and the astute parent educator, who saw himself as a citizen professional, organized a meeting with that parent to see if there was a possibility of something like a cultural messaging initiative similar to the one on overscheduled kids. (The cultural links between the two issues—schedules and parties—were clear.)

Having helped to catalyze Putting Family First, I (Bill) was able to see a path on this new initiative: Assemble a group of leader parents who would conceptualize the problem, develop cultural messaging, and try out new approaches in their own families. We met for a year to bring the project to the public stage. In 2006 we held a large launch event with the support of local parent education program, and we made use of media contacts of Putting Family First and the University of Minnesota. The launch event with 150 parents was like a pep rally covered by ABC's *20/20* and many local media outlets. My university's media relations department trained the leader parents in how to talk to media, and they signed on based on their comfort level with media interviews ranging in difficulty from print interviews to recorded TV interviews to live TV and radio call-in shows. My department at the university also helped us create a website where people could tell their stories and rate their local community on how balanced or pressurized it felt about birthday parties. A reduced version of the website is still available at https://www.birthdayswithoutpressure.org.

The upshot was that my College of Education and Human Development website nearly crashed because of volume the day after the launch event, and the larger university servers had to take over. There was a 3-week firestorm of media interviews from all over the United States, Europe, Asia, and Latin America. (Our initiative was even mentioned—and made fun of— by Jay Leno on NBC's *The Tonight Show*.) After the intense media interest subsided and the web traffic slowed, the leadership group decided that we had accomplished our purpose of stimulating a cultural conversation, and we celebrated the end of our project—with a party.

In terms of impact, the Birthdays Without Pressure Project did not have a singular new phrase like "overscheduled kids" whose visibility could be tracked via Google Books Ngram Viewer. However, it contributed to a trend toward simpler, lower stress birthday parties (e.g., Simply Well Balanced, 2022, is an available option for parents). Understood alongside Putting Family First, this project shows the power of parents organizing to counter toxic cultural messages that come in the disguise of what is best for children.

Play It Forward!

Whereas Putting Family First aimed at counteracting overscheduling at a broad cultural level, the Play It Forward! Project focused on what families could do in their neighborhood to plan and carry out family group activities that would promote life balance and child health through obesity prevention. With University of Minnesota colleague Jerica Berge taking the lead and me (Bill) providing support, we approached the mayor and the city parks and recreation director of Burnsville, Minnesota (a town outside Minneapolis). The mayor was regarded as a leader in community engagement. Our goal was to get their buy-in and to identify a neighborhood for a possible project. They recommended the Paha Sapa neighborhood because it was a dense neighborhood with many families who had participated in city parks and recreation programs in the past.

The director of parks and recreation sent emails to families in the neighborhood inviting them to a launch event where we inquired about whether child health and life balance were pressure points for this community. (They were.) We then made the case for parent leaders to come together via the citizen health care approach to design and carry out a project that would bring families together in joint activities to address those pressure points. We ended up with a leadership group of 12 members.

Similar to how the Putting Family First group began its work, the Play It Forward! team interviewed parents and youth in the neighborhood about their concerns and interests. The results were a clear desire for more neighborhood-based physical activities that were intergenerational, informal, and even spontaneous, as opposed to child-focused, highly structured, and scheduled long in advance (they didn't want one more thing to put on their calendars!). The interviews also identified local resources for such activities, including parents who knew how to organize specific sports and business owners who were willing to help advertise and contribute resources.

The leadership group then developed specific plans and went back to community members to see if the plans fit their interests. Following this consultation process, the group initiated these action steps:

- biweekly intergenerational physical activity events at local parks. These events involved informal and often spontaneous play led by local community members with skills and interests in the specific physical activities promoted at each event.

- incorporating messages about physical activity and healthy eating at each event.

Using community-based participatory research methods within the framework of citizen health care and with the assistance of a small research grant that provided interviewers and qualitative data analysts, the leadership team evaluated the Play It Forward! Project with in-depth interviews of 25 families with 6- to 12-year-old children who participated in the activities and a comparison group of families in a nearby neighborhood. About 60% of the participants were White and the rest mostly African (Somali) or African American, and the majority were lower middle class to middle class. Parents in the leadership group were also interviewed. The focus of the evaluation was on feasibility, process, and satisfaction. The published report, coauthored by members of the leadership team (Berge et al., 2016), suggested that the intervention had good community uptake and that participants in both the leadership group and the biweekly activities were highly satisfied. More than half of the families attended 75% of the Play It Forward! Events, and 33% of families attended all the events.

The Play It Forward! Project ended after several years when the parent leaders' children aged out of intergenerational play. What I learned for citizen health care was that parents can organize at the neighborhood level to address pressure points they feel in common.

6

THE CITIZEN FATHER PROJECT

In this chapter, we describe a project with men from a very different world from that of highly resourced families dealing with overscheduling and hyper-competitiveness (see Chapter 5). The Citizen Father Project with urban, low-income, unmarried fathers began about 8 years after Putting Family First and the Family Education Diabetes Series, at a time when our model was maturing. It became a proof point for the appeal and feasibility of citizen health care with a broad range of people and communities.

ORIGIN OF THE CITIZEN FATHER PROJECT

The Citizen Father Project emerged as an initiative of the FATHER Project, an agency in south Minneapolis that has worked since 1999 with low-income fathers (mostly men of color) who wanted to reconnect with their children, become economically stable, and in some cases get legal help. (The FATHER Project is now sponsored by Goodwill–Easter Seals Minnesota.) When I (Bill) was approached by the agency's executive director Andrew Freeberg to have

https://doi.org/10.1037/0000378-007
Becoming a Citizen Therapist: Integrating Community Problem-Solving Into Your Work as a Healer, by W. J. Doherty and T. J. Mendenhall

coffee, he said he had heard about other community initiatives we had been working on. He was particularly interested in the leadership development aspects of citizen health care because he noticed that some men who succeeded in the FATHER Project—went through the educational steps of the program, earned their high school equivalency credentials, reconnected with their children, and stabilized their lives—seemed to not want to leave. They came to reunion picnics, showed up at the program center just to visit and see what was happening, and proudly wore their FATHER Project t-shirts in the community.

Now this is an interesting conundrum for a social service agency. These men had completed the 14 steps in the program and were ready to become successful alumni. And they didn't want to leave! But like nearly all social service programs, the FATHER Project could offer them little more than an advisory group that met occasionally to offer input into programming delivered by staff.

This scenario struck me as a waste of human resources. I realized for the first time that social service programs for the most part have no version of the 12th step in Alcoholics Anonymous, that is, no organized way for participants to give back, no way to contribute to the mission of the program that served them, and no way to transition from client to citizen. I was inspired by the opportunity to create a way for these fathers to become agents of change.

In this conversation with Andrew, I described a potential project involving a leadership group of fathers meeting regularly and developing a way for men to contribute to the mission of the FATHER Project to support and empower low-income unmarried fathers. In subsequent conversations with him (a White professional and founder of the FATHER Project) and program director Guy Bowling (a Black man with a background as an unwed father and a lot of experience working with urban, low-income men), we worked out the criteria for who to invite. These criteria included men who had succeeded in the FATHER Project, who appeared to have the respect of their peers as shown in classes and support groups, and who seemed enthusiastic about the larger mission of the program beyond their own situation. Program staff would then invite the nominated men to come to one of two consultation meetings during which we would lay out the vision of what we decided to call the "Citizen Father Project" and see if there was potential buy-in.

To say that the group was enthusiastic would understate the response. There was a palpable hunger to give back to the program, to other fathers, and to the community. These men were honored to be among the 15 or so who were invited to consult on whether the project was viable and worth doing. About 12 of them signed up to come to a subsequent orientation meeting to get more details and make a decision about joining. My role would be to coach Guy and Andrew as process leaders and citizen professionals, to develop the meeting agendas, to take notes, and to be the keeper of the democratic model.

THE FIRST MEETING

At this point in the book, it may help readers to see what an initial meeting of a citizen health care project looks like. As shown in Exhibit 6.1, the first meeting, with Guy Bowling facilitating, opened with a brief overview of what led up to launching the project and what we hoped to accomplish in this opening meeting. Next came introductions and a question that invited the men to share their personal experience as fathers and their involvement in the FATHER Project. Then I explained the model and the frequency of meetings, after which we engaged the group around two community questions, which served as the transition to deliberating as citizen fathers:

- What barriers do fathers in this community experience in becoming positive, involved fathers? and

- Which of these barriers can fathers overcome if they work together to make a difference?

Notice that these are "we" questions addressing larger forces affecting many fathers in the community and solutions that would involve collective efforts. The men in the group readily listed community barriers—legal, economic, cultural, and others. They thought the cultural barriers—including stereotyped attitudes toward fathers, internalized negative perceptions of mothers and fathers alike, and reluctance of men to seek help—were most ripe for working on together. These men were fully aware of institutional barriers such as the legal requirement for unmarried fathers to seek access to their children via the courts (Behnke & Allen, 2007), but changing laws would be outside of the expertise and resources of this group. What they could maybe move the needle on was how people in their community saw the place of fathers in the lives of children.

MISSION, VISION, AND ROLES

The heart of the Citizen Father Project, as is true of all of our citizen therapist initiatives, is the combination of the "I" and the "we"—leveraging personal experience for the good of others in the community. Over more than a year

EXHIBIT 6.1. Agenda for the First Meeting of the Citizen Father Project

4:00 p.m. Food sharing, mingling, greeting, and orientation

- This is the first meeting of the Citizen Father Project—which will be a way for fathers who have done well in the FATHER Project to organize and give back to the community.
- There were two consultation groups, which were called together to see if this seemed like a good idea.
- Describe the criteria for inviting men to this meeting.
- The purpose of this meeting is to get everyone on board with the purpose of the Project and with how we will work together. By the end of the meeting we hope that everyone can make a decision about whether they want to be involved, and that we will have some initial ideas for the Project.

4:25 Brief Introductions: name, kids (ages, gender), and involvement in the FATHER Project

4:35 The Personal Question: What challenges have you had to overcome in order to become a positive, involved dad?

- A minute of silent reflection
- Each takes 2 to 3 minutes (say you will time and raise your hand gently when 3 minutes are up). We will have lots more time to talk in the future, so this is a warm-up; you don't have to say everything.
- Ask for a few men to say how it felt to hear the others say what they said. Just brief comments here.

5:20 Summary of the citizen health care approach and how we will work together

- Say that the group will meet every 2 weeks to plan a Citizen Father initiative that will reflect these principles.

5:30 The Community Questions:

- What barriers do fathers in this community experience in becoming positive, involved fathers?
- Which of these barriers can fathers overcome if they work together to make a difference? Everyone has a moment to reflect. Answers pooled in brainstorming fashion.

5:50 Ask who's on board for the Project and who wants to think it over and decide later, or knows now it's not a fit.

5:55 Set date for next meeting

6:00 End

of meetings, the group developed a mission, an analysis of the problems that unmarried fathers of color face, a plan of work to tackle these problems, and a set of messages to bring to fathers, mothers, and youth.

The mission of this group, developed and debated over several meetings, was framed as "Fathers working together to support, educate, and develop healthy, active fathers, and to rebuild family and community values." The vision: "Fathers changing the image of manhood and fatherhood in the urban community and beyond." We then went on to define a *citizen father* as a man who is dedicated to his children and works to build a community that supports and develops healthy, active fathers. Every word in these statements was discussed and debated in light of the life experiences of men in the group and what we all wanted to communicate to the world.

Notice that I am using the pronoun *we* because, as a citizen professional, I was part of this group, sharing my own thoughts as we went around the circle to harvest viewpoints. (My main rule was to never go first in responding to a question on the agenda.) In fact, the *we* pronoun became central to my coaching Guy as the principal facilitator/process leader of the group. I realized that Guy was sometimes saying something like this: "Here is a question I would like you guys to ponder and share as a group." Something did not feel right to me about this language in terms of the model we were using. We were all participating in answering the questions on the table when the questions were about public or community issues or about what we were going to do as a group. We were cocreating this project as a group of eight to 10 citizen fathers and three citizen professionals (who happened to be fathers too).

Even though he was a highly experienced facilitator, Guy struggled to stop saying "I" and "you" in the group. I was finally able to explain it this way: Whenever you say "I" and "you" to the group, you are outside of it, helping its members with their project. As an experienced support group facilitator, Guy realized that support group members were clients seeking personal help, so the language of "I" and "you" made sense, as in "I'd like you to think about what you are going to work on this week." But this was a citizen action group and we were all cocreators of a public-facing project. There were no providers and clients in this space, although there were differences in terms of the citizen fathers having more expertise about the current lived experience of unmarried fathers and the professionals having more expertise about group process and the model we were using.

My conversations with Guy about language are an example of what Tai and I have come to see as "model moments," times when our citizen health approach comes into greater clarity. In this case, the clarity was about the role or "hat" the citizen professional is wearing in particular situations: a therapist or service provider hat when helping clients achieve personal goals or a citizen professional hat when partnering with fellow citizens to build something for the good of many.

CHALLENGES ARTICULATED BY THE CITIZEN FATHER GROUP

The group dug deep to articulate the challenges facing low-income, urban fathers, many of them men of color, in becoming healthy, active fathers. The categories that emerged were fathers themselves, mothers and fathers together, and the larger social system. In this section and the ones following, I present the exact lists developed by the group rather than paraphrasing anything myself. I urge you to read through the lists and take in the meaning and tone of the language, which was thoughtfully developed and served as guideposts for the project. I start with the challenges facing fathers in Exhibit 6.2, then continue with mothers and fathers together in Exhibit 6.3.

The group first articulated a powerful list of challenges they and other fathers face in this community. Loss and lack of knowledge stemming from loss are major themes. The men talked a lot about how the absence of fathers in their own lives made it hard to know what to do when they became fathers. They were making up manhood and fatherhood on their own, often

---

EXHIBIT 6.2. Challenges Facing Fathers Themselves

- No "father backbone" from our own fathers—someone to push us, to stay on top of us, and to show us how to be a father
- False ideas of manhood
- Lack of manly values about taking care of babies you make and looking out for your family
- Lack of healthy relationships with our own parents
- Lack of forgiveness of our own parents
- Ignorance about the importance of dads beyond their money
- Lack of information about our own stories, such as what happened that made our dads (or moms) absent
- No tools to stay the course with a girlfriend
- Ignorance of fathers' rights
- A system that automatically gives mothers legal rights; fathers have to fight for theirs
- Many fathers don't want to go to court and so they give up
- Men being isolated from one another, unable to talk about what they are facing in trying to be good fathers

---

EXHIBIT 6.3. Challenges From Mothers and Fathers Together

- Mothers' attitude of "I can do it myself"
- The couple breakup leaves some mothers wanting to punish the father
- Mothers keeping the kids away, saying the daddy doesn't care—so the kids stop caring
- Mothers picking certain days when we can be a dad
- Mothers not being "updated" about changes that fathers have made
- Men not understanding what women go through as mothers
- Ineffective communication and conflict resolution between mothers and fathers
- Doing wrong by women creates a cycle that comes back on us and our daughters

with poor role models about masculinity and a larger system that gives them few rights. And they knew that they had few models of healthy male–female relationships beyond some of their grandparents who had stayed together for life. The last point on the list in Exhibit 6.2—isolation and not having other fathers to relate to—was a spark toward the action steps the group would eventually take.

I want to convey that these conversations about challenges were uplifting, not depressing. The group had a sense that we had to look squarely at the problems in order to create messages to counter those problems. The personal stories of father absence and sometimes of abuse by fathers connected directly with motivation to make a difference for other fathers and children.

Exhibit 6.3 addresses challenges affecting fatherhood that come from mothers and fathers themselves as they relate to one another. These were among the most delicate conversations in the Citizen Father Project because some of the men had still-fresh wounds from feeling blocked by mothers from being involved fathers. The first five of the eight challenges reflect what the group felt were mothers' contributions to them losing their children when the couple broke up. When the group went deeper, led by a couple of members who had done a lot of work on themselves with their attitudes toward women, they added challenges that men cocreate with women. The last one is particularly powerful: the cycle of how wronging women comes back on fathers and their daughters.

PLANNING FOR PUBLIC ACTION

After laying out the challenges, the group went on to brainstorm solutions they could tackle. A prelude was a discussion of the community dimension of fathering, which sets the stage for community action. The material in Exhibit 6.4

EXHIBIT 6.4. The Community Part of Fathering

- Grandchildren not knowing their grandparents–this is part of the cycle we must break.
- Fatherless families mean that daughters grow up without healthy ways to relate to men–they become too close or too distant.
- We share the same stories as the community.
- We can show the community how to make it better.
- We don't have to recycle, we can break this chain, we can make it better.
- There is a need for good fathers to be role models for others in the community.
- There is a need for personal and collective healing; unless we deal with our insecurities, we pass them on to our kids.
- We lost our roles as men in our community; we have to find our place again.

is both descriptive and aspirational: what's going on at the community level and how we wanted to change it. It was a way to articulate the larger "we" dimension of change: "We don't have to recycle, we can break this chain, we can make it better."

Criteria for Selecting our Public Action

A crucial stage in citizen health care projects occurs when the group is ready to choose its action steps. We've learned that it's important to discuss criteria for choosing action steps before brainstorming specific action ideas, some of which would otherwise end up off the table after much debate because of unarticulated assumptions about what would fit and not fit the goals and resources of the project. We've learned that people bring implicit criteria for evaluating whether an idea is good or bad, feasible or unfeasible, and it's better for a group to have explicit criteria. For example, if a group has no monetary resources (beyond, say, small expenses from an agency for food or transportation), an action idea that would cost a lot of money would not fit the criteria and thus not be worth extended discussion. Similarly, an action idea that mainly involves professional resources would not fit the citizen health care model that the group has been using. In that light, here are the criteria the Citizen Father group agreed on. Some I brought from other projects for this group to consider, and others were generated directly by the group.

- The project should aim to improve the lives (current and future) of fathers, children, mothers, and grandparents.
- It has to involve fathers "returning the favor" to the public—passing on what we've received and giving back.

- It should appeal to common ground among fathers no matter what their individual challenges.
- It should be solution focused, not just problem focused.
- It should appeal to mothers—something they would see as positive, even say "Wow!"
- The action should be visible to the community.
- Success should not depend on public officials making new policies.
- Movement forward should not require a lot of outside resources.
- Members of our Citizen Father group should have energy and passion to work on it.
- The action should culturally fit the community we are addressing.

I recall that a key criterion was the one related to mothers: that they should see what we do as positive, as something to be enthusiastic about. Ours was not to be a "fathers' rights" approach that pitted fathers against mothers.

Our Action Project and Approach

After more than a year of personal storytelling and deliberation, the group came up with two action ideas:

- reaching out personally through presentations to lots of community groups, including fathers in the community, incarcerated fathers, single mothers, youth groups, faith communities, professionals, radio, and other community groups; and
- a video documentary that uses personal stories to educate the community about problems and solutions and to give visibility to the Citizen Father Project.

We agreed to start with presentations to community groups. (The video was something the group hoped might happen eventually after implementing the community outreach work if we were able to attract the interest of a documentarian.) We then took many meetings to deliberate on how we wanted to approach the community presentations. We decided that the presentations should have the following characteristics:

- Be personal and public: our own stories and community stories, our personal solutions and community solutions
- Communicate how we feel about our children
- Let fathers know that we are here to support them wherever they are

- Offer challenges and solutions

- Push back against the stereotypes of urban men and fathers

- Inspire people but keep it real; no exaggerated stories

- We can have different roles: presenter, storyteller, singer

- A consistent message, over and over, no matter who is presenting

- Different messages and approaches for different groups: for example, for kids who may not have a father in their lives, for fathers who feel regret about not being with their children or anger at the mother, for mothers who are angry but may be open to forgiving and giving the father another chance

- Overall, the right messages to the right people: fathers, mothers, children, community members, and professionals

THE GROUP'S MESSAGES

A highlight of the group's work was the messages that we conveyed in presentations to fathers, mothers, and youth. First, to fathers.

Our Message to Fathers

- We believe that children need fathers.
  - Every child deserves a dad.
  - As fathers, we want to be important to our children.

- We believe that it takes a man to be a good father.
  - Just because you have children doesn't mean you are a father.
  - You have to be healthy to focus on your children rather than yourself.

- We believe we can learn to be good fathers.
  - Give them your time; schedule them in.
  - You can learn what it takes to be a good father even if you didn't have one.

- We have to relate to women better for the sake of our children.
  - We have to listen to them and respect them.
  - How do we want our daughters to be treated by men? Be that man.

- We believe it's urgent.
  - If you wait too long to be connected to your child, it can be too late.
- We believe this is a community problem that needs a community solution.
  - We as men have failed our children, our families, and our society.
  - We need citizen fathers who are dedicated to their children and work to build a community that supports and develops healthy, active fathers.

Our Message to Mothers

Developing messages to mothers proved more difficult and time-consuming than did developing messages to fathers. Men in the group processed their own histories and current relationships with the women they had had children with. We decided to start with the overall goal for these presentations and then address special issues in the approach to the presentations.

The goal was to change how women who hear presentations perceive men as fathers and offer hope for the future. The approach required "straight talk, compassionate talk, and future talk." This came from the group's sense that many of the mothers have been hurt and abandoned by men, don't trust men, and don't know what a healthy relationship with a man would be like. In the words of the group, "There are deep wounds, and many women have gone cold stone hard to men." Based on this deliberation, here are the messages for mothers:

- Children need fathers, and every child deserves a healthy, active father.
- It's mainly the responsibility of men to be good fathers and to promote healthy, active fatherhood in the community.
- Most men want to be the best father they can be, but they often didn't have a father in their lives and don't know how to be a father themselves.
- We know that many men have fallen down on their responsibilities as fathers and have left mothers to raise children alone. That's something we want to change.
- Mothers often hold our families together and raise the next generation of boys who will become fathers and girls who will choose the fathers of their children. That's why we need your help.
- We know that many women don't trust men, often for good reasons. We want to understand better what mothers have gone through so that

we can support them and work together to raise the next generation of fathers and mothers.

- We know that we can't be the best fathers unless we know how to have good relationships with women.

- We won't solve the problems of our communities today until we solve the problem of fatherhood. Can we work together?

Our Message to Young Men

The group knew it wanted to reach the younger generation, especially young men. This required adjusting the messages as follows:

- Fathers are important in the lives of children.
  - Every kid deserves a dad.
  - Being a good father is something we can learn how to do.
- There are good and bad times to become a father.
- Best time to become a father:
  - When you're with one woman, married and stable
  - When you're finished with your education, have a job, and are financially ready
  - When you are ready to sacrifice
- Worst time to become a father:
  - Right now
    - You lose your teen years.
    - You will be broke, and you will lose things that you will never get back.
  - When you're still living with your own parents
    - You're putting parenthood on them because you can't handle or juggle everything.
  - When kids are having kids
    - Kids don't know how to take care of themselves.
    - Kids don't understand the burden of the responsibility.
  - If you think that having a child will make you become responsible and change you for the better, think again: It's not an easy task.
  - Fathers are important to society. There is a crisis in our communities because fathers are not stepping up as fathers.

– We won't solve the problems of our communities today until we solve the problem of fatherhood.

THE CITIZEN FATHER PROJECT IN THE ACTION PHASE

Consistent with how the group developed its mission, vision, and messages, we began to do community presentations in a quite deliberate way by videotaping the initial ones and reviewing them to critique and improve the presentations. The group divided up into teams of four or five for scheduling the presentations, with Guy Bowling serving as the process leader for the panels. Each man told his own story and shared a subset of the message points, and then there was interaction with the audience.

As I attended and observed the presentations, several features struck me as distinctive features of the approach we were using. Generally in presentations by professionals and agency clients, the professional describes the work of the agency, articulates the public or community dimensions of the issue, and then turns to the client to present a success story about the work of the agency. The client tells a personal story of before-and-after involvement with the services of the agency. Audience questions tend to focus on the agency's work, with maybe some questions for the clients about their own situation.

All good, but strikingly different from Citizen Father presentations where the men tackle the public dimensions of fatherhood in their community as well as tell their own stories. To repeat: The citizen fathers handle both the public and personal dimensions of the problem and its solutions. (Guy's role was mainly facilitative, plus briefly describing the services of the FATHER Project and how the Citizen Father Project fits into the mission of the agency.) Seeing this was another "model moment" for me: It's only a citizen professional–citizen therapist project if the lay project leaders are prepared to speak to the public dimensions of an issue in addition to their own experiences.

These were among the most powerful presentations I have witnessed in community settings. I will profile the messages of Jamie (name changed), a Black man. He began by describing his terror upon learning, at age 15, that he was to become a father by an older girl and how many years it took him to come to grips with how to be a presence in this child's life. He later had more children during a time when he was living on the edge of the law, fortunately never being convicted of a felony and doing hard prison time. Lost but wanting to make something of his life and not repeat his own father's mistakes (his father was abusive before abandoning Jamie), he was referred by the state child support agency to the FATHER Project, which helped him turn his life around. He reconnected with his children through first engaging constructively with their mothers (some of whom he sadly admitted he had treated poorly). He earned his high school equivalency credential and secured a decent paying job while starting his own small business. He came to grips with the role that anger and hurt played in his life. "Hurt people hurt people," he liked to say.

In the Citizen Father presentations, Jamie would tell this story and tie it into a larger picture of men who felt lost when they became fathers in a world where many people thought they had nothing to contribute except child support, which they struggled to provide. Like the other men who presented, he made a strong personal case for what men can be for their children if given a chance and if willing to take hold of their responsibilities.

No doubt the most powerful part of Jamie's presentations when women and mothers were present was an honest admission of how he had not appreciated the mothers of his children, often blaming them for his own failures as a father. And then he would say something like this,

> I have tried to make it right with the mothers of my children. At one point in my journey to being a good dad, I realized that I had to try to make things right with my exes. I decided to approach each of them with an apology and flowers, accepting responsibility for my past actions and asking them if they would start again as coparents for the sake of our children. They all accepted. Now I want to say something to the women here. I know that men have hurt many of you in the past and that you did not get an apology. So today I'd like to apologize on behalf of men who have wronged you. I am so sorry for what you've gone through. I know this doesn't make it better, but it's from my heart.

There were few dry eyes in the room.

The presentations end with a ringing call for all of us in communities to rally around the idea that all fathers are called to be good fathers and that we can support them in that goal, for the sake of their children, the mothers, other family members, and the entire community. Although resources have not allowed for a systematic evaluation of the impact of the presentations, written evaluations by those attending have been uniformly enthusiastic, and the informal feedback has been gratifying to the citizen fathers and the FATHER Project staff. One indication of success has been the continued interest in the community for more than a decade to have the citizen fathers present.

THE PROJECT TODAY

As of 2023, the Citizen Father Project continues in its 13th year, having survived the COVID pandemic, and has returned to live presentations. The group has done more than 170 community presentations to a variety of audiences, from high schools to parent programs to staff at nonprofit agencies to prisons. There have been multiple generations of Citizen Father leaders in the group as older members move on, although two have been there from the beginning, along with Guy Bowling, who handles the booking of presentations and facilitates the group's meetings. The Citizen Father Project also led directly to the development of the Police and Black Men Project, a story we tell in Chapter 9.

7

BRAVER ANGELS

Counteracting Political Polarization

Political polarization is arguably the biggest problem facing the United States in the first third of the 21st century because it has paralyzed our government, divided citizens against one another, and kept us from solving almost all other social and economic problems (Hetherington & Weiler, 2018; Klein, 2020; Mason, 2018). Polarization has been rising for several decades across multiple administrations in Washington, DC, and it's occurring in other democracies in the world as well (Bertoa & Rama, 2021).

This divide is not so much about differences in political viewpoints (left vs. right) but about what social scientists refer to as *affective polarization, social polarization,* or *sectarianism*—in other words, how we view the large number of fellow citizens who vote differently from us. In an important review paper published in the journal *Science*, Finkel et al. (2020) summarized the three core elements of today's polarization: (a) othering (those on the other political side are alien and incomprehensible), (b) aversion (they are unlikeable and untrustworthy), and (c) moralization (they are bad people). Affective polarization has invaded nearly every aspect of American life, from local schools to Congress, from friendships, marriages, and families to national membership

https://doi.org/10.1037/0000378-008
Becoming a Citizen Therapist: Integrating Community Problem-Solving Into Your Work as a Healer, by W. J. Doherty and T. J. Mendenhall

organizations (Klein, 2020). Drastic declines in trust for one another and in social institutions has become a major characteristic of contemporary American life (Clark & Eisenstein, 2013).

In this chapter, I (Bill) tell the story of a project focused on depolarizing relationships between conservatives ("reds") and liberals ("blues") in the United States. The work began in December 2016 after the presidential election of Donald Trump and led to the founding of the national nonprofit called Braver Angels.[1] This organization, which is led by reds and blues in equal proportions, has become a national leader in addressing the problem of polarization, with members and workshops in all 50 states and with extensive media coverage that advances its message.

This chapter describes the origin and development of Braver Angels, with special attention to the workshops it offers, and its initial impact. I will connect some key decisions in the outreach of Braver Angels to citizen therapist principles. Braver Angels is unique among the projects described in this book because it is national in scale and because there are immediate opportunities for therapists to become involved in their local communities.

HOW BRAVER ANGELS LAUNCHED

About 10 days after the 2016 election, a time when I felt depleted about political engagement, I received a call from my New York City–based colleague David Blankenhorn, with whom I had worked on projects related to marriage and family life (including one where we brought together same-sex marriage advocates and religious liberty advocates). David told me that when he'd talked with our mutual colleague David Lapp, they saw a stark contrast in how their communities were responding to the election: Blankenhorn's Upper East Side Manhattan neighborhood was in shock and grief, whereas most people in Lapp's small town in southwest Ohio were celebrating a national rebirth. (Blankenhorn supported Clinton, and Lapp, although a religious and political conservative, had voted for a third candidate instead of Trump.) On an impulse, they decided to invite 10 Hillary Clinton and 10 Donald Trump supporters in southwest Ohio to spend 13 hours over a weekend to see if they could talk with each other instead of about each other—as concerned citizens and not as enemies.

---

[1] The organization was originally called Better Angels from the Lincoln phrase "the better angels of our nature." However, another organization claimed trademark protection for the term, which led to the replacement name "Braver Angels."

My first reaction was enthusiastic: We need this as a country, something local with real people and not what we were seeing on our favorite siloed TV channels. But when I asked Blankenhorn about the plan for the weekend workshop, he said that he didn't have much of an idea beyond getting people in the same room and talking. I froze, thinking about how counterproductive or even disastrous this could be without the right container for the conversation. I quickly checked my calendar for that weekend, halfway hoping that I was booked! I then gingerly asked if I might be useful in designing and facilitating the weekend. That's actually what the two Davids had been hoping for. After the phone call, I wondered what I'd gotten myself into. The workshop was 3 weeks away. Only later did Blankenhorn tell me that his New York colleagues, some liberal and some conservative, had unanimously warned him against doing this gathering—it would be a disaster, they firmly predicted, because emotions were too raw right after the election.

Lapp recruited the workshop participants from his circle of Republicans and from outreach to the county chair of the Democratic Party. The final group ranged widely in age and educational levels, and politically each side ranged from moderate to fervent red and from moderate to fervent blue. Most were White European Americans except for an African American woman (a blue), a Latino man (a red), and a woman who defined herself as a Muslim American (a blue). Interestingly, when Lapp talked to potential participants on the phone about what would happen at the workshop, people on both sides said it would be difficult because their own side dealt in facts and logic, whereas the other side was mainly about emotion.

I drew on everything I knew about group process and couples therapy in designing the workshop, which was held in a church basement (more on Braver Angels workshop designs later). The goals were that we

- better understand the experiences, feelings, and beliefs of those who differ with us in today's politically polarized environment;
- see if there are areas of commonality in addition to differences; and
- learn something that might be helpful to others in our community and in the nation.

The room felt tense before we started as people kept to small groups with others they knew. Table tents had people's names in red or blue ink. But when they responded to the opening question about why they came to the workshop, my confidence increased: They came because they were concerned about the division in the country and their community. As one group member said, "We have children to raise here, hospitals to maintain, roads to build. We can't do this if we just keep fighting each other."

Just as good couples therapy depends on creating a structure where two people at odds can listen to each other without interrupting and flaring, I knew that the success of this workshop depended on a workable structure or design. I once saw Oprah Winfrey lead a conversation on *60 Minutes* with a group of reds and blues who seemed similar to those who came to the South Lebanon workshop. With Oprah doing little more than floating questions such as "What do you think about Russian collusion in the election?", the group quickly polarized as people interrupted and talked over each other, neither side conceding an inch. When asked at the end what they were taking with them from the conversation, one person said, "We're heading for a civil war."

Contrast that with a curiosity activity we did in South Lebanon, where each side got to ask questions of clarification of the other side, with no retort or "correction" of what people said in response to the questions. The questions people asked of each other elicited commonalities based on a deeper understanding, as opposed to standard talking points. All of this was carried out with firm facilitation guardrails to keep people on track with the process (something they had agreed to at the outset of the workshop). A central learning was that they were closer than they had thought on core values and aspirations for the country and its people, while they differed (sometimes a bit and sometimes considerably) on what policies would lead to those common goals (e.g., that everyone should receive good health care and education). The process helped us to humanize each other instead of stereotyping (or demonizing) each other. Of course, this group consisted of people willing to give their time to a process of bridging the political divide, but they were not all mild-mannered centrists. Several of them routinely lit up their Facebook accounts with diatribes, and there were some intense and difficult moments during the workshop.

A document that group members discussed and signed afterward contained this summary paragraph:

> None of us, as a result of our conversations together, have changed our minds about which candidate for president was the better choice in the 2016 election. But we have changed our minds, at least a bit, about each other. We learned by talking to each other that we aren't as divided as we thought and that we aren't as incomprehensible to one another as we thought. (Braver Angels, 2017, p. 16)

At the end of the weekend, there was a sense that we had all been part of something extraordinary. Going into the experience, I had imagined it as a one-off demonstration of what was possible—and then I thought I would go back to my other work. But my closing words at the workshop portended the path I would choose: "At the beginning of our time together, I felt the pain of our nation. Now I feel the hope for our nation."

FROM A WORKSHOP TO A NATIONAL INITIATIVE

The two Davids and I realized that we had to keep going. The question was how. Would the three of us do similar workshops around the country as a sign of hope for depolarization, or would we develop briefer and more practical variations on the workshop (briefer than a weekend) and train a lot of people to moderate them? The second option prevailed because we all believed that there was something scalable here that could rally many Americans to the work of depolarizing our country.

With this in mind, I went back to Minnesota and designed 3-hour and 6-hour versions of what we called the "red/blue workshop" and tried them out locally. A key breakthrough for scalability was a decision to not screen participants the way we had for the first one in Ohio (where Lapp had personally talked with each one on the phone to orient them and make sure they were a good fit). I knew that this time-consuming step would severely limit the spread of the workshop, but I was uncertain about whether people coming "off the street" through local advertising would be willing and able to follow the ground rules and participate constructively. I took the plunge by asking a local library branch to advertise and sponsor a 3-hour workshop that contained some of the core activities of the 13-hour workshop. The result was gratifying, even exhilarating: Unscreened participants could handle the workshop activities well, and their reactions were uniformly positive. One participant, a Black Democratic activist who later became a Braver Angels leader, described the experience as life-changing. She told me and others, "Before that workshop I knew the political positions of conservatives, but here I learned the 'why' behind their views."

(Note: Over more than 2,500 Braver Angels workshops, we have consistently found that people willing to give their time do not come to disrupt, and we have had no "attack" incidents that initial skeptics of this work predicted would happen. Most of the blues did not think that Trump supporters would act reasonably, and vice versa. However, I believe that if we did not use a structure with firm guardrails, many of these same participants would act like those on *60 Minutes* with Oprah.)

We now had potentially scalable workshop offerings but no plan for how to take them to the nation (not to mention having no funds for that effort). Then lightning struck in the form of a National Public Radio (NPR) interview, which is worth discussing here from a citizen therapist perspective. My expertise as therapist opened the door. Kerri Miller, a local Minnesota Public Radio call-in radio show host, had interviewed me many times about family issues—my day-job professional expertise. In January 2017, after she interviewed me about a family-related topic, I mentioned the Ohio workshop. She immediately lit up and asked me if I could get two people from that workshop to appear with me on an upcoming national, call-in NPR show that would air during the first 100 days of Trump's presidency. She was to be the host for Thursday nights with this national audience.

The live radio show aired in early March with me and two Ohio workshop participants, a red and a blue who had become friends and could put human faces (voices) on what had happened. Afterward, something unexpected ensued. Invitations came pouring in from around the country: "Please come to our town, we'll recruit participants and find a location, and we'll help you find a place to stay." These invitations led to a bus tour in the summer of 2017 where we rented a bus and gave workshops throughout Ohio, New England, and the mid-Atlantic states, attracting people eager to join forces with us and a lot of media interest. A key learning from the NPR "lightning strike" is that our clinical expertise, if we are willing to be publicly visible, can give us legitimacy and trust that open doors for citizen therapist initiatives.

Some additional decisions reflecting citizen therapist principles were crucial to the initial success of Braver Angels. One concerns the level of expertise required to lead the workshops, which expanded beyond the initial red/blue workshop to include a variety of skills and other kinds of workshops for bridging the political divide (see Exhibit 7.1 for a list and description of Braver Angels workshops). A traditional professional approach would have been to limit moderators to licensed or otherwise credentialed professionals. Instead, I used the criterion of real-world experience facilitating small groups. This meant that we could recruit a wide range of professionals, including business and ex-military people who had led teams, organizational consultants, and lay people who led parent–teacher association meetings for a number of years, chaired school boards in rural communities, and facilitated groups in their religious congregations. In terms of workshop design, I decided to ensure that the workshops could be conducted by moderators of good but modest-level skills. This required some changes from the original workshop exercises that took every skill I had, and even then I sometimes broke into a sweat!

The point is this: If you want to scale a civic intervention across the country in a short time, cast a wide net for leaders and make the offering doable without graduate-school training. Other modifications also aided the scaling of the workshop. For example, I learned that participants need more support to frame good questions of understanding for the other side. In the first

EXHIBIT 7.1. Braver Angels Offerings

Experiential Workshops

Red/Blue Workshop

Brings together equal numbers of conservatives and liberals to better understand the influences on one another's political beliefs and to look for common ground. Carefully designed to build trust and foster increasing openness between the groups over the course of the workshop.

Everyone is welcome, but this workshop is incredibly vital for people with homogeneous ideological circles who may be looking to broaden their perspective.

Each online session lasts about 3 hours. In-person events include either half-day or full-day formats, with half-day workshops including the exercises from Session 1 and full-day workshops including both sessions.

Session 1. Get beyond the stories we tell about each other to discover the truth, and create a forum to discuss our viewpoints without judgment.

Session 2. Go further in the search for common ground by asking sincere questions of understanding and getting real answers. Discuss actions we can take to move this work forward as individuals and as a group.

Common Ground: Single-Issue Workshop

An outgrowth of the signature red/blue workshop, this workshop allows participants to go deeper into a single issue, setting up a foundation for joint action. By developing points of agreement on values, concerns, and policies, groups can identify potential actions to advocate on an issue, such as op-eds, shared speaking engagements, and meetings with community and political leaders.

Skills Training Workshops

Teach participants skills that can be applied within their existing relationships and in a variety of settings, extending beyond purely political conversations. Participants come from all walks of life, but these programs are particularly helpful to those already dealing with relationship stress over politics.

Skills for Bridging the Divide

Learn techniques to speak with those you disagree with so you can be heard, listen in order to truly hear, strengthen relationships, and find common ground.

Depolarizing Within

Recognize your inner polarizer, and affirm the value and humanity of the other side, even among people you agree with. Intervene in polarizing conversations without risking accusations of disloyalty or naiveté.

Available as either a hybrid eLearning course and live workshop or a 2.5-hour fully live session combining instruction and practice with partners.

Families and Politics

Learn skills for handling family political differences in a constructive way while remaining true to one's values and political beliefs. Recognize the unique risks that come with political disagreements between family members and the different roles family members can play in those discussions.

(continues)

EXHIBIT 7.1. Braver Angels Offerings (Continued)

Skills for Conversations About Race and Public Policy

This workshop offers skills and perspectives to help participants listen better to people who have different views on the public policy dimensions of race in America, express their own views in a constructive way, and seek common ground when it is present. The workshop exposes conservatives and liberals to the principles and beliefs of the other side on issues such as affirmative action, policing, and reparations, and gives them tools for navigating conversations across these differences.

Other Events and Experiences

Braver Angels Debates

Parliamentary-style debates designed to encourage freedom and clarity of speech, mutual respect in disagreement, and a shared search for truth.

May include any audience, but particularly engaging for academic settings. Braver Angels has a special college debate program to bring in younger members, which has vastly increased its presence on college campuses in the past year and a half.

Also a very effective tool to bring in red participants, who often gravitate toward debate-style events.

1:1 Conversations Across Differences

A novel way for different types of people to connect personally as concerned citizens, to understand each other's experiences and beliefs, and to discover commonality and bridge differences. Available between red-blue, urban-rural, person of color-White, and intergenerational pairs. Each format includes two structured 1-hour conversations between two people using an online video call.

Ohio workshop I'd had to intervene to help people reframe gotcha questions before the other side responded. (One participant got reactive when I tried to change her question, and I had to use my therapist skills to calm her and keep her from leaving the workshop.) So, I changed the design to have the red and blue groups meet with separate moderators to spend 20 minutes coming up with four good, curated questions—a learning process for each group and a process that led to better questions and less need for a moderator to have to intervene in real time during the question-and-answer exercise.

The second decision informed by citizen therapist principles was that we would train moderators without charging them a fee and would expect them to deliver the workshops without compensation. The traditional professional model assumes that professionals will pay considerable sums to get trained and certified in a new model, after which they recoup their training costs and enhance their incomes by providing the new professional service.

In Braver Angels we decided that this approach was inconsistent with rapid scaling of the workshops at a time of national need. Instead, we envisioned a large cadre of citizen moderators doing this work, not full-time or as part of their income plan, but as a way to give back to their country and empower its citizens.

The third decision caused more disagreement among the emerging group of Braver Angels leaders: how to do the moderator training. We began by offering several daylong moderator trainings on the East Coast, attended mostly by people who lived nearby. I did those training workshops in a traditional way: presentation, video demonstrations, and question-and-answer session. I realized several things after three trainings: They were too dependent on me flying around the country, live events would involve considerable travel expenses for trainees who did not live in large metro areas (thus limiting the rapid availability of the workshops in less populated areas), and they were one-time trainings delivered in a "fire hose" way that did not really allow trainees to return to the material (other than via a manual). And any thought that in-person trainings with 30 people allowed me to assess their competence was an illusion. On the latter point, the supposed advantage of in-person training is quality control of who would do the workshops—something that would require multiple sessions and observations of trainees doing workshops, elements that were not possible within the resource constraints of Braver Angels and without charging considerable fees for the training (in other words, without using the traditional professional credentialing model that leads to relatively few trainees going through a time-consuming and expensive funnel to full certification). For example, we wanted someone in a small state like Idaho who had facilitation experience to be able to train right away and start doing workshops without having to first fly to a big city for a training session scheduled months in the future.

The upshot was that we decided to offer future moderator training in pre-created online modules, extending to about 15 hours and including full-length videos of me moderating a red/blue workshop and one of the skills workshops. This self-paced training would be followed by a live, online orientation wherein an experienced moderator and I would meet the new moderators and answer their questions. In 2022, when we had a larger number of experienced moderators who were interested in helping with moderator preparation, we added a requirement that the trainee do an online demonstration of the ability to describe and manage one workshop exercise.

I sound more confident now in the Braver Angels moderator preparation approach than I was at the time. It was scary to abandon the traditional model of making sure that moderators had professional-level credentials and in-person training. How would such a varied pool of moderators handle these workshops? I told myself that the worst outcome of poor moderation was likely a negative experience trying to depolarize and a confirmation of participants' current stereotypes of the other side. "This is not brain surgery," I told myself, and the participants are not distressed clients seeking mental health assistance.

When the first cohort of trained moderators began doing workshops, I held my breath until I started receiving consistently positive postworkshop evaluations from participants, along with informal feedback from workshop organizers who were present at every workshop (no moderator is alone with a group). I was mightily relieved. Evaluations were consistently strong across a range of moderators—and have been for over 5 years. When an occasional moderator is not good at the task, they usually know it and take on other roles such as organizing workshops for other moderators. Local workshop organizers, too, invite the better moderators for future workshops. Bottom line: I felt I had succeeded with workshop designs that could be competently delivered by people with various backgrounds. Note that the moderators are neutrals when doing the workshops: They do not identify as red or blue even if they do have a political leaning.

A final step toward Braver Angels as a national-level initiative came after a 2017 retreat where the leadership team decided to form a nonprofit membership organization that would be half red and half blue in leadership at every level and that would rely primarily on citizen volunteers to carry out the work of depolarization and not on paid professional staff. The main job of staff would be to empower and facilitate the work of regular citizens, along with fundraising and representing Braver Angels to media and other organizations. On my end, I was a volunteer allowed and encouraged by my university employer to devote time as part of my public outreach work.

THE BRAVER ANGELS WORKSHOPS

As mentioned, in designing the workshops I borrowed from everything I had learned about group process and communication skills since my graduate-school days in the 1970s. I had learned a lot from the Public Conversations Project (later Essential Conversations), which was founded by family therapists Laura Chasin and Dick Chasin (Chasin et al., 1996). The original aspects of Braver Angels workshops have come from applying couples therapy principles such as (a) the importance of moderators intervening rapidly to enforce the structure and prevent escalating and hijacking the process and

(b) eliciting expressions of humility about the contributions of one's own side to national problems.

Exhibit 7.2 contains a description of the exercises in the cornerstone red/blue workshop. The participants are five to eight reds (defined as leaning conservative and generally voting for Republicans) and five to eight blues (defined as leaning liberal and generally voting for Democrats). There are two moderators. (As mentioned, they do not have to be a red and a blue because moderators are neutrals.) After goals are presented, ground rules explained, and introductions made, the group begins with the stereotypes exercise: In separate rooms, reds and blues are asked to come up with the four most common false or exaggerated negative stereotypes that others have of their side (the stereotypes they think others have about them, not the stereotypes they have of the other side). Then each group goes through the stereotypes one by one, answering two questions: "What's true instead (in other words, correct the stereotype)?" and "Is there a kernel of truth in it?"

Reds' most frequently self-identified stereotypes are that they are racist, xenophobic, heartless toward the needy, antiwoman, antiscience, and Bible thumpers. For blues, most common are arrogant or elitist, into big government for its own sake, fiscally irresponsible, encouraging of dependency, unpatriotic, antimilitary, and baby killers. Note that the workshop intentionally begins by getting out on the table the worst things that each side thinks of the other but in a process that encourages each side to acknowledge the stereotype and gives them an opportunity to correct it without being attacked by the other side. For example, reds get a chance to express their commitment to human equality across all races despite their concerns about specific policies related to race as well as their concern for the needy along with their wish that local sources of help predominate, when possible, as opposed to federal bureaucratic sources that can encourage dependency. Blues get a chance to say that they believe in fiscal responsibility while holding that spending money to create equal opportunity saves money in the long run and that criticism of one's country is an essential part of patriotism.

The "kernel of truth" question is a key one in the workshop. It's a chance to express humility and show a balanced perspective about one's own side. Moderators tell the group that kernels of truth might take the form of something that is true of a subset of people on one's side, was true historically, reflects a blind spot or something not paid much attention to, or stems from how one's side comes across in the heated rhetoric of public debate. Examples of red kernels of truth from workshops include the regrettable presence of racists on their side and the reality that some of their leaders denigrate immigrants. Blue examples include acknowledging that some blues

EXHIBIT 7.2. Red/Blue Workshop Exercises

1. Stereotypes Exercise
   - Red and blue groups meet separately to come up with five false, exaggerated, or misleading stereotypes of their <u>own side</u>. In other words, what do others get wrong about your side? This is a chance to correct false stereotypes as well as to acknowledge any kernel of truth in them.
   - They go through the stereotypes and decide how they are wrong and what is true instead of their side. The moderator writes down these points.
   - For each stereotype, the moderator asks for any kernels of truth: for example, true of a subset of their group, had some truth in the past, reflects a blind spot, or heated rhetoric in public debate may contribute to the stereotype.
   - The whole group regathers and someone reports out from each group, with the moderator helping to make sure the summary is clear and covers the kernels of truth as well as the corrections of the stereotypes.
   - Reflection question afterward for the whole group: What did you learn about how the other side sees themselves, and did you see anything in common?

2. Fishbowl Exercise
   - One group sits in a circle responding to questions while the other side sits in an outer circle to listen and learn. No interaction between the inner and outer circles. The goal is to learn about the other side without the expectation of responding.
   - The two questions: (1) Why do you think that your side's values and policies are good for the country? and (2) What are your reservations or concerns about your side?
   - Then the circles switch positions.
   - Reflection question afterward for the whole group: What did you learn about how the other side sees themselves, and did you see anything in common?

3. Questions for the Other Side Exercise
   - Each group meets separately to generate four questions of understanding for the other side—questions to clarify and go deeper rather than gotcha questions intended to challenge or catch people in contradictions.
   - The facilitator helps the groups curate their questions to reflect the goal of more understanding, and everyone writes down the four questions word for word.
   - Then reds and blues combine into two mixed groups where they take turns asking each other the four questions and can also ask follow-up questions.
   - These exchanges are tightly facilitated in order to stay within the guideline: only questions rather than inserting one's own opinion.
   - Reflection question afterward for the whole group: What did you learn from the questions exercise we just did?

4. Action Steps Exercise
   - Participants fill out an Action Grid with ideas for what they can do individually, what they can do with others from their side, and what both sides can do together to promote understanding across the political divide and find common ground—in a larger way, to prevent long-term civic divorce.
   - They share what they came up with in red/blue pairs.
   - Then they share a highlight with the whole group.

come across as arrogant and elitist and that blues sometimes go immediately to large government programs without necessarily asking how effective current programs are.

While each group works on the stereotypes, the moderator suggests a spokesperson from the group to share these reflections with the other group. After this, in pairs and then in the whole group, a reflection question is posed: "What did you learn about how people on the other side see themselves, and did you see anything in common?" Particularly when each group has "landed" the kernels of truth, the learnings from both sides can be striking. A central feature of moderator training is to press both groups to do the self-criticism involved in the exercise.

This stereotypes exercise starts the workshop by getting the worst accusations on the table but in a safe way. It allows each side to express their core values that sometimes do not come across in public conflict, and it encourages each side to express humility about their role in society's divisions. The moderators' job in this exercise and the others in the workshop is to steer the agenda, create a space for sharing and listening, and enforce the ground rules that emphasize respectful listening and speaking. In that sense it's like being a good couples therapist: creating a safe environment for people to say what's on their minds and in their hearts and to listen deeply to each other. Couples therapy requires the ability to intervene quickly and authoritatively the moment that one partner interrupts, becomes sarcastic, or speaks for the other. In Braver Angels, the moderator has to be both permissive of people saying what they want to say (no coaching on the "right" view to express) and limit-setting (immediately redirecting someone if they veer from the question on the table at the time).

LEARNING FROM THE BUS TOUR

As mentioned, a key part of the development of Braver Angels was the bus tour through 14 towns and cities where we had a chance to fine-tune the workshops (we had only two at that point—the red/blue and a general skills workshop). Here's one story from the tour.

When our group arrived in Ithaca, New York, midway through the 1-month tour, we were tired and looking forward to freshening up, but there was no running water in the Airbnb we had rented. Things got worse in the morning when we discovered that the site for the all-day workshop was a day care center with tiny tables and chairs. Fortunately, we were able to raise the table legs. Still lacking enough adult chairs, we put in an emergency call for our local host to bring or rent chairs. (Fortunately, they arrived on time.) Later in the day, the septic tank broke and the one toilet got overwhelmed, rendering it unusable, and the septic tank repair person treated us to loud pumping sounds during the last part of the workshop.

I tried to not see a metaphor in all of this, which was good because the workshop group was exceptionally articulate and well-informed. They got into the spirit of the day with the stereotypes exercise and by lunchtime were fully on board. In fact, for the first time, I started to really take in the red perspective about how government bureaucracies gravitate toward over-regulation. Although I'm still a liberal, I found myself appreciating the value of the limited-government perspective they articulated—in another era, Thomas Jefferson was saying the same thing. I could suspend, at least temporarily, my counterarguments (say, about the inability or unwillingness of some states to address important health and social policy issues) and absorb what the workshops were about: listening to how others see themselves and seeing if there's common ground.

I'm a bit embarrassed to admit that I hadn't expected to be affected in the same way as I wanted workshop participants to be affected. My identity as a citizen therapist was shifting away from polarization, and I began to recognize an overlap between the citizen health care model and certain aspects of conservativism—such as the emphasis on local initiative and ownership of ways to solve local problems. Of course, local civic agency can be a liberal value as well, but there is often more emphasis on large government initiatives.

I was also struck by the insight of a local Republican Party official when he added this kernel of truth to the racism stereotype: "We Republicans aren't that good at looking at history and our part in problems like race and gender. We tend to stick with the point that things are better today." Then two young Republican women, who had been holding back among outspoken men in their group, did a nice job of agreeing with their fellow reds that Republicans are the party of opportunity—in that they emphasize equal opportunity, not equal outcomes—but noted that opportunity isn't always equal for women and minorities. Similarly effective was the moment when blues began to challenge each other on their party's rigid and often elitist sense of what's right for all of America.

These moments helped me realize that the major movement in these workshops came when each side showed humility and vulnerability. As in couples therapy, breakthroughs happen when each partner owns a piece of the problem rather than assuming the high ground from which to point out the other's flaws. That's why in the fishbowl exercise, which follows the stereotype exercise (see Exhibit 7.2), we ask paired questions of each group while the other group sits in an outer circle and listens: "Why are your side's values and policies good for America, and what are your reservations or concerns about your own side?" Almost always, the other group softens rather than pounces when people own up to their concerns about their own side.

A personal highlight for me happened over a meal at the end of the Ithaca workshop. A liberal Black man invited me to share, now that the day was over, whether I'm a red or blue, because he couldn't tell. A White woman sitting next to him said she also couldn't tell. Seeing my job as advocating for both sides to bring out their best selves, as I do as a couples therapist, I was gratified to hear this. If I'm even-handed in facilitating workshops, my personal politics shouldn't be obvious. Although I did tell them that I'm a blue (both of them were also blues), I took the uncertainty of these two observant people as a sign I was doing my job.

THE SCOPE AND IMPACT OF BRAVER ANGELS

From its beginning in December 2016, Braver Angels grew steadily in membership and in-person workshop participants until the COVID pandemic shut things down in March 2020, after which the workshops shifted to online formats for 2 years. There was steady momentum, particularly around the 2020 election. As of winter 2023, more than 2,500 workshops have been held, plus more than 1,000 one-to-one structured conversations that are based on the red/blue workshop (see Exhibit 7.2). A Braver Angels–style debate process, developed by April Lawson, has been conducted more than 100 times. These are cooperative, parliamentary-style debates designed to encourage freedom and clarity of speech, mutual respect in disagreement, and a shared search for truth. They have tackled the most divisive topics (such as whether the 2020 election was stolen) with a structure that allows for responsible airing of differences and careful listening for commonalities. Finally, a Common Ground workshop, developed by therapist Reena Bernards, allows participants to listen carefully and articulate shared values, concerns, and solutions on topics as polarized as abortion.

Braver Angels' paid membership is more than 12,000, there are about 600 trained workshop moderators, and there are about 100 Braver Angels Alliances, which are state and local associations of individuals who have attended Braver Angels workshops and who want to continue the conversation and promote workshops in their local area. Funding comes from membership dues ($12 per year), foundations, and private donors. Outside funding sources have been nearly evenly divided between red-leaning and blue-leaning sources. Although the general membership skews blue, there is red/blue balance at every level of leadership from the board to the leadership team, volunteer state coordinators, and Alliance membership. The ratio of volunteer leaders to paid staff is about 10:1.

Outside observers of Braver Angels have offered two main challenges to the work: (a) Are the workshops effective in depolarizing participants? and (b) What about public officials and the political halls of power—if you don't reach them, will grassroots efforts be effective in depolarizing America? On the first question, limited resources meant that for the first years the only available evaluation data came from participants completing a questionnaire at the end of workshops. Those evaluations have been uniformly positive, with self-reported learnings and attitude changes averaging between 4 and 5 on a 5-point Likert scale. It has only been more recently that Braver Angels has attracted the interest of academic researchers who want to study the effects of workshops using standardized measures of polarized attitudes and behavior. One completed study using a randomized controlled design and a 6-month follow-up found significant effects on attitudes and behavior toward the other side after a red/blue workshop (H. Baron et al., 2021). Unpublished preliminary results from an additional academic study found similar changes with the Depolarizing Within workshop (see workshop description in Exhibit 7.1). Thus, although more research is needed, we have reason to believe that Braver Angels workshops are effective in fostering depolarization at the individual level.

When it comes to public officials, we have begun to attract interest and participation in an initiative called Braver Politics. This work began informally in 2019 with skills workshops for 30 Minnesota state legislators and then a red/blue workshop for city officials in Maryland. After a pause during the pandemic, we have been approached by groups of elected officials for whom we've created specialized workshops. One of those workshops invites small groups of legislators (at both the state and congressional levels) to share their responses to this question: "What life experiences have influenced your values and beliefs about public policy and public service?" This is followed by a conversation about polarization and how to reduce it in their setting. I have been moved by responses from New Hampshire state legislators and members of Congress when we've done this activity in small groups. These officials have gone deep with the 5 minutes each is given to answer the question, followed by a question about what they learned from listening and what they found in common. They've told stories of loss (parental death, widowhood, Holocaust deaths in their extended family) and stories of inspiration (including grandparents who were community pillars and encouraged public service).

Here is a moving and enlightening example from the life experiences exercise: A Democratic legislator talked about his experience growing up in the foster care system and how it motivated him to run for office to help these kids. His story was immediately followed by a Republican colleague who said, "Wow! This blows my mind. I grew up in foster care too and it's been a driver of my career." The Democrat wanted to make a difference via government services, whereas the Republican was focused on how the voluntary sector could lead the way, with government encouragement.

A life experiences session I did with members of Congress was similarly impactful, even though cameras and journalists were present! One member talked about how the death of her beloved husband impelled her to carry on his political legacy and make it her own at a time when many were not accepting of women in politics. Another talked about growing up in poverty with minimal expectations for his life but with a mother who encouraged him to visit the state capitol with her and told him that he could serve there when he grew up. At the end, a Republican member who had told the group at the beginning, "I am conservative as the day is long," said that the take-home effect on him was the sense that "You can't fight someone in the same way when you know their heart."

Another new workshop for elected officials is called Managing Difficult Conversations With Constituents. This came out of presentations I gave for county commissioners and city officials about polarization. Their main pressure point at the local level was polarized constituents (from both sides) and people who were just plain agitated by everything going on in the world. This workshop teaches listening and connecting skills along with ways to use "I" statements in explaining one's positions and finding something to agree with, if possible. A similar workshop focuses on managing conversations with colleagues who are politically different. We teach what we call the prime directive: Connect first, then share your view. County commissioners, mayors, city council members, and school board members have responded enthusiastically and given the workshops strong evaluations. We hope that our political science research partners will do more systematic evaluations in the future.

HOW CITIZEN THERAPISTS CAN GET INVOLVED

Braver Angels has opportunities for graduate students and practicing therapists to contribute to the work of national healing and depolarization. You can take workshops offered locally in person or nationally online and then train to moderate workshops. You can join and provide leadership to state and local alliances that serve as follow-up groups for people who have taken workshops. You can help organize workshops. You can become a Braver Angels ambassador who gives presentations in local communities about the problem of polarization and what we can do about it. You can help with Braver Angels research and evaluation.

One reason that citizen therapists can be especially useful in the work of depolarization is that we are accustomed to self-reflection about our own biases and emotional reactivity. In that light, the application for becoming a Braver Angels moderator offers the following for self-reflection for applicants:

> This work is about depolarization, and that can be very emotional. We need people who have respect for the other side and who won't respond to getting their buttons pushed by someone of a different political persuasion. In the moderator role, you must be neutral and you have to create a space where everyone feels respected, where everyone in the room says that the moderator wasn't emotionally reactive to either side or wasn't trying to "correct" either side. You cannot see the other side as deplorable or ignorant or deserving of pity. You would have trouble doing this work if your goal is to "enlighten" the other side. In short, you cannot be emotionally triggered by people who have political views that are very different from your own.

WHAT THIS WORK HAS MEANT TO ME

On a personal level, my citizen therapist work with Braver Angels has been among the most challenging and rewarding experiences of my career. In terms of challenges, working closely with Braver Angels leaders who think very differently from me about politics and public leaders has meant that I have to deal with a kind of diversity not much discussed in the therapy field, namely, political and ideological diversity. I have had to let go of my stereotypes about conservatives and have come to recognize my own blind spots.

As for other challenges (and in the spirit of Braver Angels humility), I want to describe what I worry about for the organization and its work. I worry about the imbalance in membership (3:1 blues to reds) even if we have balance in leadership. I brood over the fact that our membership and workshop participants are mainly White and upper middle class. (We have a red caucus, an "angels of color" caucus, and a working-class group, but who knows if they will change our membership profile.) I fret about whether we will burn out volunteers who devote 30-plus hours per week and about whether our fundraising will allow us to retain a large enough staff. There is more money in polarizing issues than in depolarizing. I worry that future leaders of the organization, after its founders move on, will succumb to the gravitational pull of a traditional professional organization where all decisions are made centrally and regular volunteer citizens are helpers but not leaders. May it not happen!

I also sometimes struggle to hold hope that this work can succeed. Polarization seems to have gotten worse since we started Braver Angels, and the events on Capitol Hill on January 6, 2021, nearly knocked me off my horse. I worry about potential civil unrest and even an insurgency or civil war, events that seem outside of the scope of what Braver Angels could help with. There are large forces at play in the land, and many conflict entrepreneurs are stoking the fires of division. Recently other Braver Angels leaders and I have concluded that Braver Angels will succeed only if we help to stimulate a social movement embracing many segments of society. We will not workshop our way out of this mess; a new initiative is about forging partnerships with other groups and organizations who also fear for our country.

The rewards, too, have been enormous. I have formed deep civic friendships with people working for the common good, and my learning about political worldviews besides my own has grown exponentially. Moderating the workshops is always uplifting. But most of all, I feel immense satisfaction that I get to use my skills as a citizen therapist to respond to the gravest national crisis of my lifetime.

PART **IV** PROJECTS
DEALING WITH
RACE

8 THE RELATIONSHIPS PROJECT WITH YOUNG BLACK MEN

In this chapter, we describe a project involving young Black men in Minneapolis who were enrolled in a high school class taught through the Office of Black Male Student Achievement in Minneapolis Public Schools. The Relationships Project offered an opportunity to see how our citizen professional work could be extended to a population of teenagers who were grappling with the twin issues of racism and the academic achievement gap (Kuhfeld et al., 2018). Would these young men take to a democratic, disciplined process that emphasizes personal and collective agency in making changes they initiate on their own? To foretell what becomes clear later in this chapter, the answer was an enthusiastic "yes," although the project had a premature ending when a budget crisis hit the school system.

ORIGIN OF THE PROJECT

We've learned in our citizen therapist work that one project often opens doors to another one. In this case, Bill's work with the FATHER Project involved his doctoral student Corey Yeager, a Black man with considerable experience and

https://doi.org/10.1037/0000378-009
Becoming a Citizen Therapist: Integrating Community Problem-Solving Into Your Work as a Healer, by W. J. Doherty and T. J. Mendenhall

skill in working with young Black men. When Corey was hired as a consultant to the Office of Black Male Student Achievement in Minneapolis Public Schools, he approached the office director Michael Walker with the idea of using the citizen health care approach with students taking the B.L.A.C.K. course (signifying "Building Lives Acquiring Cultural Knowledge") at South High School, a class for which Corey and Michael had been leading a weekly support group.

I (Bill) recall well the first coffee shop meeting with Corey and Michael when they talked about how this group of students wanted to go deep in understanding and dealing with the challenges they faced in their multiracial school that had mostly White teachers and administrators. The question for me was whether the model that Tai and I were using could add value to the good work already being done with these students. We are both White and had never worked in school settings, although Boyte's public work model (see Chapter 1, this book) had been used extensively in a school-based project called Public Achievement (Boyte et al., 2018). I recalled Tai's phrase when we come upon possible new ventures: "Have model, will travel."

In that coffee shop I spun out an idea based on two principles of my clinical and community work: agency and relationships. What about a project that focused on two key relationships that no doubt influence these high school students' learning in school—relationships with teachers and young women? Current efforts to improve academic achievement among Black students were addressing other important issues, including developing a proud Black identity through learning Black history, mentoring and tutoring from Black professionals, getting peer emotional support, and in-service training for teachers. Relationships could be a potential innovative area, that is, students working on their relationships with teachers and young women to enhance their experience and learning in the school. We would use our democratic method in which the professionals would be process leaders and the students would take responsibility for coconstructing the project at every phase.

Corey and Michael said they were in. We agreed that they would be the process leaders, and I would coach them on the process, develop meeting plans, and take notes during meetings. The key next step was to meet with the 18 students in the class to see if they would buy into the idea and the approach. The students were mostly juniors and seniors, many of them from low-income families. We posed two questions for their consideration:

- Are your relationships with teachers an important part of your learning and success in school?

- Are your relationships with young women an important part of your learning and success in school?

The responses were strongly affirmative. A key point in their responses to the first question was that if they had a poor relationship with a teacher, they felt unmotivated to learn the material and succeed in the class. (Research supports their observation [Legette et al., 2022]). And given a poor relationship, they were hesitant to approach the teacher for help when they fell behind. A key point they made in responding to the second question was that of distraction from "girl drama" in their relationships, which made it hard to focus on learning in school.

We thus had an agreement on the importance of these two relationships for academic success. At this point a traditional professional approach would be to develop a curriculum to teach the students how to interact better with teachers and young women. There is nothing wrong with this approach, but it's not a citizen professional way of working. It's not cocreative.

Instead, Corey and Michael asked me to explain the citizen health care way of tackling the goal of better relationships with teachers and young women. Here is a summary of what I said:

- We've shown one another how important these relationships are and that they can be challenging and difficult for being successful in school.

- The basic idea: This group takes the lead to develop a project to empower Black male students to change relationships with teachers and young women for the better—not asking the teachers or young women to change at this point but showing that we will take the lead to have better relationships.

- The approach emphasizes people facing a challenge by taking the lead in solving it, using democratic decision making, going deep before taking action, spreading what we learn to other young Black men, and being both bold and practical.

The students were inspired, even fired up. They were ready to start. However, because this launch meeting occurred in April, the school year was going be over in a couple of months, which meant that we would be setting the groundwork rather than doing the whole project. It was then that I realized there would be a turnover of more than half of the students for the following fall. This occurred each of the 3 years of the project, which meant that we repeated some version of the buy-in process with each new group consisting of some returning students and new students. Fortunately, the word got out that this was a cool, engaging project, and we were able to navigate shifting group members (sometimes from semester to semester as well during a given academic year).

THE FORMATIVE STAGE OF THE PROJECT

Because we've learned that the first few meetings of a citizen action group are crucial for creating the culture of a project, we offer details about the meetings of the Relationships Project following the launch meeting. Near the beginning of the second meeting of the Relationships Project, we reviewed, clarified, and revised what the group had offered about relationships with teachers and girls at the launch meeting. Here are the final versions the group agreed on.

First, on how relationships with teachers affect our school success:

- Relationships with teachers can make the difference between doing the work and succeeding—or failing.

- It's hard to have a good relationship with a teacher who we think stereotypes us.

- It's hard to have a good relationship with a teacher who carries over a negative attitude toward us after one bad experience in the classroom.

- When we're angry about being treated unfairly or disrespectfully, it's hard to show respect and do the work the teacher asks of us.

Second, how relationships with young women affect our school success (at this point, the group was using the term *girl* but later shifted to *young women* after getting feedback from other students):

- We get distracted from academics.

- These relationships are draining.

- [There is] a whole set of emotions to deal with.

- The wrong girlfriend can lie, spread rumors, and hurt our other relationships.

- It can be hard to take care of a girl and focus on school too.

- We can attract the wrong girls—and be attracted to them too.

- The right girl can make a positive difference in how we succeed in school.

- It's best that school be first, girls second.

Once we had agreed on the relationship challenges we wanted to work on, the next step was to have a consensus on how we would work together. Corey and Michael proposed the following principles, which the group deliberated about and agreed to. We read these principles aloud at each subsequent meeting of the project:

- We focus on what we can do ourselves, on our end, to improve relationships with teachers and girls. We go first in making changes.

  (This was the key norm of the project, the way the group kept a focus on personal and collective agency instead of emphasizing what others—especially teachers—were doing wrong and how they should change.)

- We take time to go deep.

  (This norm created a context for deliberating at length and in depth before taking actions that could be premature.)

- We think big and act practically.

  (In citizen therapist projects, this is how we frame a big vision beyond the immediate group and project while doing concrete actions.)

The following set of ideas and practices emerged over the next few meetings as we reflected on our group process and larger purpose:

- We are disciplined in our group process, including not having side conversations, not using cell phones, and limiting interruptions. We hold ourselves accountable in our meetings.

  (This created a standard of conduct for the group, not always upheld in practice because these were energetic and sometimes distracted adolescents, but something we returned to regularly to reinforce the norms the group had agreed to.)

- We will develop strategies for improving relationships with teachers and girls—for us individually and for other African American young men in this school and beyond.

  (This one in particular inspired the group.)

- We will emphasize what we can do ourselves, on our end—and then see how teachers and girls might change in response to our changes.

  (This is an elaboration of the first principle. Notice how the hope for others to change is included here but as a subsequent step after personal initiative by the students.)

- We will work democratically, and with discipline.

  (This one emerged from a discussion about what a democratic process looks like—everyone's voice counts—and the need for discipline in our process in order to make democracy work.)

THE TEACHER RELATIONSHIPS PART OF THE PROJECT

The group decided to work on teacher relationships as the initial action priority, given that teachers were an identifiable group who could be approached in a school setting. (Young women in the lives of the students could be in this school or elsewhere.) I proposed that the group interview teachers as a prelude to deciding on action steps to improve those relationships and that we begin by articulating the values we want to bring to relationships with teachers—and get feedback from teachers about these values. This made sense to everyone.

The Values We Want to Bring to Relationships With Teachers

A powerful part of the project was generating the values the students held for their relationships with teachers. We brainstormed a list of values and then discussed and debated each of them at length before coming to consensus. Here is the final set of values the group said they want to bring to relationships with teachers:

- Honesty and integrity—being real, not fake
- Respect—offer it and hope for respect in return
- Trust—seek their help and hope they will be fair
- Commitment—going to school and doing our best
- Communication—speaking up and asking for help
- Patience—listen to their point of view
- Don't stereotype them—just as we don't want to be stereotyped
- Love—treat them like parents

The process of developing and discussing these values was profound for me. (I teared up as I typed them here.) The values confirmed that these young men were not approaching problems with teachers just from a position of grievance and complaint (although there was much to grieve and complain about) but from a stance of agency and empowerment. They immediately embraced something that therapists usually only learn during training: In relationships we can only control our own part and our own behavior and then hope that the other will respond constructively.

I want to highlight three of the values. Students in this group often felt stereotyped by teachers (there are few groups more stereotyped in our culture than adolescent Black men; Taylor et al., 2019), and yet they articulated the value of not stereotyping teachers, particularly White teachers "just as we don't want to be stereotyped." This is the Golden Rule applied by a group with less power to a group with more power. A second value, trusting enough to seek help, came from soul-searching conversation. The students were aware they had internalized male norms of not showing weakness by asking for help. They knew that they had to get past this attitude if they were to succeed academically, which meant being vulnerable with teachers. (This may have been the biggest change group members made in the project.) Finally, "love—treat them like parents" was the subject of much discussion and revisiting over the 3 years of the project with each new cohort of participants. Was this something to aspire to? Was it realistic? At the end of each deliberation, the consensus was to retain love as a value.

The First Action Step: Interviewing Teachers

The goal of the one-to-one teacher interviews was to learn how to improve relationships with teachers. The whole group generated a list of teachers to interview, beginning with ones considered friendly. They individually invited teachers with a written note and did the interviews in pairs, with one asking the questions and the other taking notes. The interviews had three parts:

- sharing the goal of the interview,
- asking several questions that focus on what we can do positively to improve our relationships with teachers, and
- sharing our values and how the teacher thinks we can show them in relationships with teachers.

See Exhibit 8.1 for the handout given to the teachers at the start of the interview. It has the questions and the flow developed by the group over several meetings. The students found these interviews a rewarding experience, interacting with teachers in a different, initiative-taking way. They felt proud about going public with the Relationships Project. On their end, several teachers told the students how impressed they were with the interview. (One teacher said it was the most powerful experience of his teaching career.) Teachers resonated with the values articulated by the students, although one teacher had an interesting response to the question about how students can take the initiative with teachers: She thought relationship building was only the teacher's job, not the student's. (Not a citizen professional perspective!)

At each weekly meeting (all held during class time) the students reported on their interviews and answered questions from the group. Then we generated the following themes from the teacher interviews, framed as input for developing good relationships with teachers:

- Get to know the teacher as a person, find something in common.
- Be honest about who you are as a person, including your problems.

EXHIBIT 8.1. Interview Handout for Teachers

1. Our goal in these interviews is to learn from teachers about how you think African American male students can improve relationships with teachers.

2. These interviews are part of the Relationships Project that aims to promote the academic success of Black male students by improving our relationships with teachers and young women.

3. The approach we are taking is to learn what we can do ourselves, on our end, to improve these relationships—and then see how teachers and young women might change in response to our changes.

    Question 1: In your opinion, how can African American male students have a good attitude in class?

    Question 2: What are the three most important things African American male students can do to improve relationships with teachers?

    Question 3: How can African American male students initiate a relationship with you?

    Now we'd like to share with you the values our group decided we want to bring to our relationships with teachers. You can take a moment to look at them, and then we'll read them out loud. (Note: See the values list above.)

    Question 4: What do you think of these values, and how do you think we can better live them out in our relationships with teachers?

    Question 5: Our final question is: What is your dream as an African American male student?

    Do you have any questions for us?

- Talk to the teacher regularly about "school stuff."
- Sit in the front of the classroom.
- Do your work in class.
- Ask for help.
- Assume that the teacher wants the best for you.

Actions to Improve Relationships With Teachers

Now it was time for the group to generate specific ways they wanted to build better relationships with teachers. This took several meetings to discuss, debate, and refine. We were guided by reading our mission, focus, and values at the start of each meeting. (We read these aloud in the circle to help ground us in what we had already developed.) After agreeing on 10 actions, we categorized them into "direct schoolwork actions" and "other relationship actions." In the "direct schoolwork actions" category were the following:

- Getting to class on time
- Getting our class work and homework done

- Taking the class seriously: listening well and asking good questions
- Asking for help during and after class
- Talking about what we want from the class, including grades we are aiming for

In the "other relationship actions" category were the following:

- Building a relationship: being honest, having conversations before and after class
- Approaching the teacher with respect
- Not arguing with the teacher in class; don't ramp up a conflict—just stop talking
- Repairing relationships by apologizing and explaining
- Expressing gratitude

The first four actions could be considered standard "good student" behavior (such as showing up and doing the work), a way to fulfill the student's part of a learning relationship. They would appear on any list of ideal student behavior. The subsequent six actions were less traditional and more inherently relational. Some were proactive: talking about goals for the class, proactively engaging the teacher before and after class, and being respectful. One was preventive: avoiding escalating conflict by pulling back from arguing. The last one, "expressing gratitude," made the list after considerable discussion about whether teachers should be thanked for doing their jobs. Was this being fake? The conclusion was that teachers are human beings doing a hard job, and they deserve gratitude especially when they have something extra for a student.

To help students focus on a specific relationship with a teacher, we handed out a form that they filled out and handed in (see Exhibit 8.2). They identified a teacher with whom they wanted to improve the relationship and rated it where it currently was and where they would like it to be by the end of the semester.

Weekly Consultations

Once the students had articulated what they wanted to work on with teachers, we created a group consultation process in which students would ask for time to get input on something they were doing proactively with a teacher or on how they could respond to a challenge they were experiencing with a class and a teacher. Initially the presentations usually began with a complaint about a teacher, say, for not being clear about expectations or treating a Black student different from White students or not handling a conflict well

EXHIBIT 8.2. Worksheet for Agenda Setting With Teachers

THE RELATIONSHIPS PROJECT
IMPROVING RELATIONSHIPS WITH TEACHERS

Your Name: _____

Think of one of your current teachers where there is room to improve your current relationship.

Teacher's name: _____

Rate the relationship right now on the following scale (from 0 = *terrible* to 10 = *perfect*)

Current relationship (circle a number): 0   1   2   3   4   5   6   7   8   9   10

Now indicate where you would like to take the relationship by the end of the semester.

Circle a number: 0   1   2   3   4   5   6   7   8   9   10

---

with the student. Sometimes other students would start to weigh in on their similar experiences with this teacher or another one.

These moments were where the norm of "we go first in making changes" came into play. Corey or Michael, after empathizing with the student's distress, would remind the student and the rest of us what we had decided. I recall Corey saying to a student, "Who can you change in this situation? The teacher or yourself?" The student replied, "Myself." Then Corey would say, "That's how we agreed to work here: We focus on changing ourselves and then hope that the teacher will shift in response to our changes. We read this at the start of every meeting." Without fail, the student would change course and begin to reflect and ask for input on how he could better respond to the teacher. Over time, the group internalized the norm, and members would invite each other to reflect in this way.

I want to make it clear at this point that we did not see student initiative as a solution to all the problems that created the achievement gap. The school was doing teacher training in understanding and countering implicit and explicit racism. The B.L.A.C.K. class itself focused on self-empowerment via appreciating Black history and culture. However, group members consistently said that the Relationships Project gave them a sense that they could create and own an initiative to improve their key relationships in the school.

Examples of Consultations

A major change many of the students wanted to work on was to ask for help from teachers. A common pattern was to fall behind in a class, feel helpless about making up ground, and then be invisible in the class. One day, Jamal (not his real name—all names mentioned in this section are disguised) asked for consultation time to tell the group a success story in which he tried different behavior. Taking his cue from two of the action steps, he approached his math teacher after class and told her that he wanted to earn a higher grade in the class and asked her for her input on how to get there. The teacher was delighted and offered to meet with him after class on a regular basis to help him toward his goal.

In another consultation, Derrick began by complaining that one of his teachers was biased because she reprimanded him more frequently for the behavior (talking, clowning around), and she did not come down as hard on White students for doing the same things. Group facilitator Michael responded, "Maybe that's true. But let me ask if it's also true that you're fooling around too much in that class." Derrick agreed that he was. "So, your choices are either to challenge the teacher for being biased or to change your behavior so that the teacher doesn't have a reason to come down on you. Given what we're trying to do in the project, what's your choice?" Derrick ruefully admitted that it would be better for him to change his behavior. A fellow student then suggested that he approach the teacher after he had made this change and tell her that he was trying to pay more attention and not fool around in class. Derrick wasn't so sure about this latter input but said he would consider it. I don't recall the follow-up, but the consultation is a good example of how the group worked on challenges.

A more dramatic example came from LeShawn, a student with admitted emotional problems who was given to angry outbursts. (A year before he had blown up at a teacher, fled the classroom, and led the security staff into a tense standoff on the balcony of the auditorium.) LeShawn recounted a new incident that could have been as bad. In his social studies class, he had put his arm around his girlfriend. The teacher approached him and asked him to remove his arm from his girlfriend's shoulders. When he did not comply, the teacher touched his arm and asked him again. LeShawn exploded in anger (he had a particular vulnerability about being touched without his permission), "f-bombed" the teacher, and ran out of the room. He ended up in the library, where he calmed down. Recalling the messages and support of the Relationships Project, he knew he wanted to repair the breach with his teacher, whom he did like. So, after school he approached her, telling her that he was sorry for what he said to her and that she was a good, kind teacher who didn't deserve to be treated this way. He said he had an anger problem and was particularly upset when touched because of something that happened earlier in his life, but that didn't justify how he treated her. The teacher not only accepted his apology but said she had a loved one who also struggled with anger. She gave him a book chapter that her loved one had found particularly helpful. LeShawn reported all of this with pride, saying that not only had he repaired a relationship but it was rock solid now. The group cheered him.

THE YOUNG WOMEN PART OF THE PROJECT

The work on relationships with young women did not take off until the final year of the project because of the complexities of managing the teacher part with shifting cohorts of group members as students graduated or had schedule changes. As mentioned, we had to reboot at the start of each year. By the third year, however, we were ready to address relationships with young women. We generated values the group wanted to bring to these relationships and conducted focus groups after deciding that 2:1 interviews would be too intimidating to the young women. We then made a place for consultations at our weekly meetings, alongside consultations about teachers. A challenge was that some students were not in relationships (we did not ask about the sexual orientation of the students), and others had relationships not connected to the school. The result was that the discussions, while often searching and intense, were more general about male–female relationships than about particular relationships that could interfere with or help school achievement.

Despite these limitations, what the group generated was rich, as was the feedback from the two focus groups with young women, and worth documenting here. Exhibit 8.3 contains the focus group questions asked of groups of four to five young women who were invited by the students to participate. (One of the groups included the adult mother of one of the young men in the group!) It also contains the values the group had articulated beforehand. Two students did the focus group panel interviews while the rest of the group observed. I witnessed powerful responses from the young women when they were asked these open and vulnerable questions from their male peers. (They said they did not expect their male peers to act this way.) Exhibit 8.4 contains summary notes of the feedback from the two focus groups and the take-home messages. Exhibit 8.5 shows the action steps the young men committed to taking. Respect was the central theme of the values and the conversations with the young women. If the Relationships Project had continued, we had the raw material for something remarkable and productive in the future, including engaging young women more directly in the work we were doing.

EXHIBIT 8.3. Focus Group Questions for Young Women

1. What do you look for in a relationship with an African American male?
2. What are the three biggest things we can do to have better relationships with young women?
3. What are some ways that we make young women uncomfortable in relationships, and how can we change those?
4. How do relationships between young women and African American male students affect the classroom environment?

Now we'd like to share with you the values our group decided we want to bring to our relationships with young women. You can take a moment to look at them and then we'll read them out loud.

[Pause until they have read the values, then read them out loud.]

The Values We Want to Bring to Our Relationships With Young Women

Respect and appreciation
Being real, no games
Understanding where they are coming from
Communication—being clear about agendas
Taking things slow, building the relationship
Putting effort into the relationship
Loyalty
Trust
Commitment
Love

5. How do you feel about these values?
6. What suggestions do you have for us to better live up to these values?
7. Do you have any questions for us?

EVALUATION

In the third year of the project, after we felt we had the process down well, we planned an evaluation of the work on improving relationships with teachers. The process consisted of students choosing two teachers with whom they wanted to work to improve relationships. They gave those teachers evaluation forms to fill out at the beginning of the year and then again at the end of the year. The forms asked for teacher ratings of the student on each of the 10 action behaviors, listed earlier in this chapter, which the group has articulated they wanted to work on. Unfortunately, the evaluation was cut short by serious budget cuts (the teacher data were gathered but not analyzed), and the Relationships Project ended that year. Corey moved on to other employment, and Michael was not able to continue with work because of academic and administrative responsibilities. We had hoped to spread the

EXHIBIT 8.4. Key Messages From Young Women

Messages From the First Focus Group

- Respect was a main theme: how you would treat your mother
- Another main theme: not pressuring to have sex—talk about things beforehand
- Hitting a female is not okay
- Honesty and loyalty
- Not acting dumb and playing around to impress girls
- Keep your relationship problems out of school
- The values are great but don't just say them—do them, practice what you preach
- Help each other out in school
- Ideal African American male is smart and confident but not cocky
- Don't let the media influence how you see beauty in a girl

Messages From the Second Focus Group

- Respect was the biggest theme
- Appreciation, not forgetting what women are like
- Not being controlling
- Not touching when they don't want to be touched
- Not showing off in class
- The values are great
- But actions speak louder than words

Themes the Young Men Drew From the Focus Groups

- Respect was the key take-home message
- No name calling and using a smoother tone of voice; no bullying
- Sometimes they may feel disrespected even if they seem to like something we say or do
- Treat them as we want our moms or grandmothers to be treated
- Think first before saying things that might come across badly
- It can be hard to think first before acting
- We have to hold ourselves accountable; if we don't live our values out there, this is all a waste

EXHIBIT 8.5. Action Steps With Young Women

- Respect, respect, respect—in words and actions
- Taking time, building the relationship, and talking before expecting anything sexual
- Being real, no games
- Being loyal
- Keeping our relationship problems out of school
- Being mature—and not acting dumb and playing around to impress young women
- Putting effort into relationships
- Being careful about how we use social media—it can really hurt young women
- Resisting media influences on how we see beauty in women
- Motivating ourselves and holding one another accountable in school

Relationships Project to other schools, including a middle school, but that was not to be. However, a number of the young men in the project have stayed in touch with the adult leaders and sought their input and mentoring.

FINAL WORDS FROM BILL AND PROCESS LEADER COREY YEAGER

I (Bill) can attest to the enthusiasm that students expressed for the process and for the changes they saw themselves making. They took beautifully to the democratic, cocreation process and readily adopted the personal agency approach of going first in making changes. For me as a White professional, the Relationships Project was a powerful experience of being embedded weekly for nearly 3 years with a group of Black young men and two remarkable Black professionals. I played a satisfying role as bearer of the model we used, crafter of the weekly meeting process, and notetaker. I participated in the check-in and check-out phases of the meeting and occasionally offered a question or a viewpoint. The experience deeply influenced my thinking about racial equity by showing me the enthusiasm and ability of young Black men to make a difference for themselves and their peers even when forces in their environment work against them.

For me (Corey), the experience of working with these young Black men who sought to become better students and learn ways to leverage their relationships with teachers was one of the most important and meaningful projects I have had the honor of being a part of. As a relational, contextual, and systemic therapist, I found in the Relationships Project an opportunity for the culmination of skills that I have learned as a therapist. As a Black male who was simultaneously leading this citizen professional process and learning from the same process, I had my own self-discovery. Social psychologist Claude Steele coined the phrase "the burden of suspicion" that became critical to how I thought about the Relationship Project (Steele et al., 2002). Black students often enter academic settings shackled with a burden of suspicion, feeling as if a teacher or professor sees them as incapable of learning in the ways that White students do. Our students in the Relationship Project felt this burden, while at the same time the project gave them a space and a set of tools to unburden themselves of such suspicion. In our democratic process and flattened hierarchy, I too learned to unburden myself as I traversed my doctoral program. This citizen professional process offered me a useful and pragmatic approach to address the ills experienced by young Black men in the academic arena.

9 THE POLICE AND BLACK MEN PROJECT

Our community of Minneapolis has been a focal point of racial reckoning in recent years after a number of police killings of Black men. After the murder of George Floyd in particular, the nation and the world experienced a firestorm of protest, outrage, and political backlash (Dyson, 2020). This chapter describes a project that I (Bill) helped to start in the early years of this controversy. It's been the most high-pressure citizen therapist work of my career, and the experience has helped to solidify my understanding of a partnership way of working on social change in a polarized era.

ORIGIN OF THE PROJECT

In the aftermath of yet another local police shooting of an unarmed Black man in the summer of 2016, I decided to drop in at the office of Guy Bowling, with whom I had worked on the Citizen Father Project (see Chapter 6) and other citizen health care initiatives. The local community was reeling after the death of Philando Castile during a traffic stop in Falcon Heights, Minnesota—a first-ring

https://doi.org/10.1037/0000378-010
Becoming a Citizen Therapist: Integrating Community Problem-Solving Into Your Work as a Healer, by W. J. Doherty and T. J. Mendenhall

suburb of Saint Paul and about a mile from my house. Although upbeat by disposition, Guy said he was experiencing "outrage fatigue." Generally he tried to find a way to understand how mistakes on both sides—the officer and the Black man—spiraled into a tragic death. Or at least he could tell himself how to avoid being shot by a rogue officer (follow orders, don't run, etc.). But Philando Castile had done everything right and was still shot and killed as his girlfriend live-recorded the incident. I listened supportively but felt helpless: This huge social problem was outside of anything I thought I could address.

Then Guy asked if the citizen health care model could apply here. He had seen this approach bring people together to work on intractable problems. Guy had friends and family members who were police officers, and he knew many Black men who had been harassed by police. Was there any way to bring these two groups together to work on distrust between police and Black men—and hopefully save lives?

Sitting there in Guy's cramped office at the FATHER Project, I began to spin out what such a project could look like. The basic idea was that a small group of police officers and Black men from the community would meet frequently over at least a year to develop relationships of trust and then decide on joint action steps. As with other citizen health care projects, we would not know exactly what we would offer the community until we got to that stage of the work. Go deep, then act together.

How would we recruit participants? Guy and I both felt that the project should focus on men—male officers in the Minneapolis Police Department (MPD) and male community members—because that's the flash point in police interactions with the Black community. We knew that Black men from the community could be brought to the table; we were particularly interested in men who had experienced the citizen health care approach and thus would have patience with the process. But neither of us had relationships inside the MPD. I had never faced this challenge before, having neither direct ties nor a sponsor who could connect me to a community or institution. A misstep here would doom the project by resulting in hitting a brick wall with the MPD. I will go into some detail about this initial stage of the project because it offers lessons about being strategic in starting citizen therapist initiatives on controversial issues.

I decided to consult with my colleague and friend Sylvia Kaplan, who years ago had trained as a therapist and was well-connected in the Minneapolis political world. For our lunch conversation she invited another person who knew the police system. I laid out the basic idea for the project and said I needed help with where to start with the MPD. They told me that frontline officers didn't trust initiatives coming down from the police chief's office and suggested starting with the head of the police union. Officers would be more likely to consider participating in a project that had the support of the union.

I've rarely had luck sending cold messages to public figures like the union president. So I looked up his administrative assistant and called her first. I briefly summarized what I wanted to say to her boss and asked for the best way to get an email in front of him. She liked the idea of the project and told me that if I sent an email to the union head and copied her, she would make sure he looked at it. So I sent the email and immediately received a positive response and an invitation to meet Officer Dave O'Connor, a union board member and public engagement officer. Later that month I met over coffee with Dave and his police partner, who were both enthusiastic about the idea of a project where Black men and police officers could form real relationships instead of arguing about who needs to change. Dave took several weeks to vet the idea with colleagues and superiors and got green lights.

I was clarifying the pitch for the project as I went along. A key element was to bring together officers and Black community members for a long-term, cocreated project in which each group learned about the other and took joint responsibility for promoting community safety. As I looked at existing police–community relationship activities, I found that they focused on either community members telling officers how they had to change (e.g., large public meetings where police officials wore their professional "masks" as they listened impassively) or on ways for communities to better understand the worlds of officers (e.g., do ride-alongs with an officer or attend citizen police academies to see how police are trained). But a level playing field that started with relationship building? That did not seem to exist.

Now it was time to approach Police Chief Janeé Harteau. My friend Sylvia shared our idea with a city councilwoman whom the chief trusted, asking her to tell the chief that she would be hearing from me about a creative new project. Officer Dave O'Connor also paved the way by letting the chief's assistant know I would be asking for a meeting. When I arrived in the chief's office, I knew that she would give me a serious hearing because she had invited her community liaison assistant Sherman Patterson to attend (he is Black and she is White). In retrospect, I think there were two key selling points in what I presented. First, I told my own story of coming to realize that without public support, police could do little to enforce the law. This story involved being on the streets of Washington, DC, during the uprising, chaos, and destruction after Martin Luther King, Jr., was assassinated; the police were helpless to restore order until the National Guard arrived. Second, I expressed my sense of the limitations of big public meetings where people took turns at microphones berating (and sometimes defending) the police. I said that the key was not public gestures but building relationships based on mutual knowledge and understanding.

Chief Harteau was on board and assigned Sherman to work with me to recruit the officers. They were nominated by a group consisting of Sherman Patterson, Dave O'Connor, the deputy chief, and me. I had final screening authority because I wanted to have confidence that the officers would approach the project in a collegial fashion and be okay with months of relationship building. (Officers were released from their shifts to attend meetings.) Once we had a list of nominees, we met with the precinct inspectors (captains) to get their buy-in and willingness to approach the nominated officers. The inspectors were uniformly positive about the project and then recruited the officers. Guy Bowling and I recruited most of the community members (one was nominated by Sherman Patterson), and we interviewed them with Sherman. The community members were Black men from a wide range of backgrounds and education levels; all but one had experience with the citizen health care approach via the Citizen Father Project (Chapter 6) or the Relationships Project (Chapter 8). We decided that the meetings would alternate between a police training facility and a community-located facility. The rationale was to provide safe, familiar territory for each subgroup. The officers preferred the training facility to one of the seven precinct sites where some of them worked because they felt more comfortable there (they all went to this facility for training and it was considered neutral ground).

This is an appropriate place to note that citizen health care groups always make deliberate decisions about where to meet. A key element is where group members will feel most at home. For example, the FEDS program (Chapter 2) met at St. Paul's Department of Indian Work, and the SANTA Project (Chapter 3) met in a classroom rather than an administrative room.

PHASE 1: THE CRITICAL LAUNCH PHASE

The group of seven community members and six officers (four White and two Black) began biweekly meetings with this mission: to forge connections between police officers and African American men that can lead to better partnerships for community safety and law enforcement. I proposed and the group agreed to a process of building relationships through personal storytelling, opening up challenging topics, and deciding to create a common narrative to describe who we are, how we see the problem, what we envision for a safe community, and how we want act together to bring about change. We met every other week for 2 hours during the first 2 years of the project, and then monthly.

There were so many important conversations during the initial phase of the project that it might be helpful to exemplify them via a voice memo I recorded and transcribed after the third meeting (see Exhibit 9.1). At the time I was facing the challenge of establishing whether the group was willing to use the citizen health care process of disciplined structure for meetings— in other words, would they allow me to facilitate in the way I had learned is important for a group to form as a team as it worked toward creating a vision for its future work? The second meeting had not been a good example of this way of working, in part because one of the senior officers had blocked me from holding to the structure of the meeting, which was going off the agenda we had agreed to and devolved into a debate between two officers and two community members about police versus community responsibility for addressing crime. Specifically, this senior officer had told me to "let him finish" when I tried to redirect conversations or intervene when someone was overtalking. During the next 2 weeks I resolved to bring my concerns to the group in hopes that we could find a way forward that allowed me to be the process leader and the group to have enough freedom so that members did not feel stifled or blocked. (This is akin to couple, family, or group therapy where the therapist has to be in charge of the process or it will become unproductive, and the clients have to feel that they can also be themselves and speak their truth.)

As the transcript in Exhibit 9.1 shows, after we resolved what family therapists refer to as "the battle for structure," the sharing that ensued was powerful. The transcript captures the flow and content of a crucial early meeting of the project, along with my subjective reactions. I encourage you to read it before proceeding with the rest of the chapter.

PHASE 2: STORYTELLING AND RELATIONSHIP BUILDING

Over the ensuing months, we used a process of personal storytelling in which each member of the group got 5 uninterrupted minutes to answer a series of questions, followed by reflections from the group. I used the stopwatch function on my iPhone to time the sharing, going back and forth between a police officer and a community member. The questions in turn were as follows:

- What were your early life experiences with police officers?
- What were your early life experiences with Black men?
- What were your early life experiences with White men?

The goal here was to get to know one another as human beings with backstories. I participated in the storytelling so that the group could get to

EXHIBIT 9.1. Transcript of Bill Doherty's Voice Vemo After the Third Meeting

I felt a sense of powerlessness after the second meeting when the senior officer in the group (a Black man) overrode me several times when I tried to redirect or widen the conversation by saying to me, "Let him finish." Although it ended up to be a constructive meeting, I had the sense that this project could really go off the rails with too much intense debate too soon if I did not have permission from the group to manage the pace of our work.

During the past week I consulted with an experienced colleague about the group process, and I watched an MSNBC episode with a town hall meeting in Chicago with a White facilitator/interviewer, Chris Hayes, and an all-Black audience of maybe 50 people and a panel of police officers and elected officials. The town hall was chaotic, with people talking over one another and appearing to be giving the speeches they had come prepared to give, with little listening. The angriest people got the most applause, and those who spoke more moderately were met with silence. Nobody looked happy with the experience. At the end Chris Hayes said something like, "Well I'm not sure how much good this did for the people in the room, but perhaps around the country people could see how many dedicated Chicagoans are trying to deal with the issues of crime, the murder rate, and police-community relations."

Afterward I woke up in the middle of the night saying to myself that this project could go the same way and that I have to empower myself to take this by the reins and forge an agreement on a way that we could gradually grow in intensity rather than flaming out. I thought of the analogy of mph and speed limits: We have to start the group off at slow speed to build relationships, and then we can find our working speed. So I decided we had to have a conversation about a way of operating and my role as facilitator. But I was really nervous.

People came to the third meeting in fairly good moods. In the check-in one of the White police officers first said, "I'm feeling fine about our meetings," and then he said, "No, I'm not." He said last time the stories and arguments were difficult for him and made him feel hopeless. Then when the senior officer checked in, he looked at the rest of the group and exhorted them all to be honest and get to the point. He was clearly acting like the group leader and had double authority as the senior officer and the oldest Black man in the group.

When it came to my check-in, I said that I was hopeful about our work and also concerned about the process, which is why I had put the process of our group on today's agenda. I laid out my concerns, and then for a while after that things went badly from my perspective. One of the community members whom I had worked with for a couple of years in other settings responded by saying that Black people have to work too often within a kind of rigid constraint and can't really say what's on their mind, and he doesn't want to be shushed. One of the other community members (again, with many years of experience in groups with me) said, "Yeah, we are people who like to just get in there." The senior officer agreed with that.

I decided I was going to push back. I said there have to be guidelines that we agree on that I can facilitate from. Somebody said, "Well, you can throw the yellow flag if it gets too intense," and everyone laughed. I said I don't think it's going to work that well because it's going to come down to my arbitrary "referee decision" that it's getting too intense. There has to be a way that this is doable and predictable. Fortunately, one of the other community members with good group skills weighed in, kind of looking for compromise, and was joined by another community member who vouched for me and my way of leading groups. One of them said that he would never come to a series of meetings with the police as a Black man if I was not personally leading it, but maybe there needs to be some stretching of this because this is a different kind of issue and different kind of group.

EXHIBIT 9.1. Transcript of Bill Doherty's Voice Vemo After the Third Meeting (*Continued*)

I went with that compromise, and others backed away from the idea that Black people don't do group limits. We all agreed that we need a place we're weighing in with honesty but that we needed some ground rules. I proposed that if I come in with a plan for what we're going to do at the meeting and if nobody has any objections, we follow that plan. And if I felt somebody was diverging a bit too much from the original plan, I would propose we table their point or come back to it or kind of steer them. And if somebody looked me in the eye and said they wanted to finish their point, I would say, "Go for it." But I don't want third parties, other members of the group, telling me that I should let you finish. In other words, self-responsibility. I'm sure everybody knew I was implying that I didn't want the senior officer or anybody else telling me to let someone else keep talking. That officer showed a small smile as he nodded in agreement.

Then the mood lightened, and I told them that I had lost sleep because I was really worried about this, and I care a lot about this project. I then explained that my belief is that we have to build relationships as well as engage in conflict and that we do need to have some speed limits. I gave some examples that seem to help, like I said suppose somebody says that the police department's racist and somebody else says no it's not. What are we going to do with that? Now it's an important question about racism in the police department, but if we're going to tackle that one we're going to need a whole meeting to do so. We're going to need a plan, not just do it off the cuff. I would propose that let's just start with what we understand by that word *racist*. Or suppose somebody turned to a police officer and said, "What are you going to do to hire more police officers of color?" Same thing: an important question that needs a deliberate process to get into.

I added that right now we're in storytelling mode, getting to know each other, and that we will get to solutions but that this is not the time for debating solutions. They seemed to get that. I was sort of showing my own energy and power right then (this was a group of powerful people). I said I want you to know that I'm not afraid of conflict. I do marriage counseling for a living. I deal with people in conflict all the time. What I want is a place that can allow us to deal with conflict proportionate to how we have come to understand and trust each other, and we will then get to a place where I think we can come up with some really creative things for the community.

Now I was fully engaged and no longer anxious. (I could tell beforehand how anxious I was because my hand was trembling as I was trying to take notes during the check-in.) When the first few comments had not been responsive to my concerns, I had to remind myself that I brought this group together and that everyone had agreed in principle to the model I proposed using—and I don't have to stay and continue with the group if I can't feel constructive. (It's a lot like therapy in that way: I have to be in charge of the process in order for people to get something from our work together.)

For the rest of the meeting there was good honest dialogue. Some of the police officers were open and vulnerable. One said that he had not known police officers personally but went in policing to serve and to help others, not to arrest people and give them tickets. An example of feeling misunderstood was when he was on night duty in north Minneapolis. He responded to a 911 call from a woman who said she'd been hurt by her boyfriend and would someone come and arrest him. So as the officer is driving a Black man to jail, the man in the back seat keeps yelling "You just want to arrest Black men and you don't care about Black people." In his own mind the officer was saying, "Man, I just helped this Black woman who you beat up, so what do you mean I don't care about Black people?" One of the community members responded, "I wish I had known more officers like you." The officer responded that his motto, learned in his youth, is to treat everyone like they are your grandmother.

(continues)

EXHIBIT 9.1. Transcript of Bill Doherty's Voice Vemo After the Third Meeting (*Continued*)

Another officer shared that it feels like the table has been set on the north side of Minneapolis for years before he arrived. The table has been set in terms of community and police relations, and his question is whether it will be different when he retires. He felt bad that he has to ask that question, but he has to believe that there can be a change.

A community member asked an officer if his personal life ever spills over, like a bad mood or something's wrong at home. The officer replied that yes it affects him and getting grief from somebody is harder to take and your job is to just, you know, try not to let it out, but it's hard. Then he added something powerful: that police officers feel like a sponge for all the pain and distress and violence in the community.

There were moments of disconnection too. A community member complained that the county sheriff's officers did not respond on time to his 911 call related to his son who had escaped from custody, and his father (the community member) knew where his son was—by a bridge. (He feared for his son's safety.) Three squad cars went by and did not stop, and it was 45 minutes before a sheriff stopped to retrieve his son. The senior officer clarified kind of gently and calmly that they have call priorities and that if it's violence, that gets a higher priority, and sometimes for a nonviolent thing, you know, could be 30 to 45 minutes. He also said that the county sheriff's department is different from the Minneapolis police. But that response didn't mean anything to this upset father, who said, "You guys wear badges."

Then another community member shared about a past experience of being pulled over with his four children in the car and with him wearing a suit and tie. One officer was White and the other Black, and they had their guns out, accusing him by saying that there had been a robbery of a cab and they thought it might be him. The White officer said, "Are you Eddie?" whereupon the father showed him an ID badge that was connected by a bit of elastic string. The officer sneered and pulled the ID badge, letting it snap back. All of this in front of the children, with no explanation about the mistake and no apology. All very distressing as he told the story. The officers all agreed that this was a bad stop, particularly because he had his four children in the car ("Cab robbers don't wear suits and drive with their kids in the back seat") and that he deserved an apology, which would have lowered the distress of the encounter.

The senior officer then said that it was upsetting that the Black officer didn't do anything and that Black officers can be worse sometimes than the White officers. He then said something memorable: "We have some cocky cowboys in the department, and they get angry and don't know how to apologize," and so that was pretty powerful.

We ended with the check-out question "How do you feel about our work in this meeting?" Excerpts:

"I feel responsible as a man to do something."

"I enjoy seeing some of our officers out and about in the community, and I can approach them as a friend."

"When you see me on the street with my dreads, you now know me as a person who is not dangerous."

"We're starting to pull this, pull things out of the jar, you know, we've got a full jar, one at a time, and we're pulling things out and it's starting to work."

After the meeting a lead officer said it's hard to see how we're going to come up with any actions and any solutions, but he trusts that something will emerge. I replied that this process involves not knowing the end product yet, and we just have to trust that we will get there.

So, it was a really great meeting. Guy Bowling, the cofounder of the project, told me afterward that "this is very difficult, and it's historic." That's how I'm feeling at the moment.

know me. Early experiences with police officers were telling. A number of them had fathers or other relatives in law enforcement and had generally inspiring experiences, whereas most of the community members at best had distant relationships with police, seeing them as an occupying force in the neighborhood to be avoided whenever possible. When they encountered police officers, they often felt harassed and disrespected. One community member, though, shared how he was saved from a life on the streets by an officer who befriended him. The officer got him involved in learning to box, which turned him into a disciplined athlete.

We then talked about our fathers, with stories both sorrowful and uplifting. Most of the officers had active fathers, whereas many of the community members spoke, sometimes tearfully, of father absence and in some cases abuse, experiences that they had resolved not to repeat with their own children. (They also told of the surrogate fathers in their families or communities.) As I reflect now on these father stories, it strikes me that the officers, familiar with male authority figures, entered a hierarchical power with mostly male bosses—a social world quite different than that of men in the urban communities they were serving.

Another memory from this phase of our work was that I was the only White man in the room who acknowledged growing up with racist attitudes toward Black people. The N-word was omnipresent during my childhood in working-class Philadelphia of the 1950s. The White officers, on the other hand, described more tolerant upbringings and talked about having Black friends and classmates. I didn't know whether this difference was generational (they were a good deal younger than me) or whether the officers were reluctant to reveal any taint of racist attitudes in their pasts. I do recall the Black members of the group, both officers and community members, looking relieved when I talked about my early environment—it confirmed how they saw parts of the White world. I also talked about the complexities in my family when it came to race. Like Archie Bunker (a 1970s TV character), my father had strong negative stereotypes of Black people; however, he also talked about specific Black men in his work world with familiarity and affection. Everyone in the group laughed when I told the story of how my wife noted that the photos of my father's retirement party showed mostly Black men in attendance, something that my parents had not noticed and seemed a bit embarrassed about when my wife teasingly asked, "Where are the White people?"

Through these stories we came to know each other as human beings. We had some conflict during this phase of our work, but mostly we focused on building connection. We were laying the cornerstone of trust for the next phase.

PHASE 3: MORE TURBULENT WATERS

As we got into police–Black community topics, we used a structured process in which each group member had a chance to share and be listened to, with no expectation that we would reach a consensus in the short term. Sometimes we went around the group to hear everyone's voice before more general conversation. Sometimes a community member and an officer had a back-and-forth conversation, with the rest of group reflecting later on what they heard. I felt like an orchestra conductor—or more like a leader of a jazz ensemble with just enough discipline and structure to keep everyone involved and not let it descend into cacophony.

How we processed the police shooting of Jamar Clark, an unarmed Black man, marked a milestone. Before our group began to meet, Clark's killing had sparked weeks of demonstrations and an encampment outside the police precinct in the neighborhood where we met. There were heated exchanges in the group between a Black officer who had been responsible for maintaining safety during the protests and a community member who had been involved in the encampment (and who had previously led community protests). The heat in these exchanges did generate some light as the two men came to better understand each other's perspectives and found some common ground. Neither was a villain in the other's story.

PHASE 4: PROCESSING NEW EVENTS

A counterpart of meeting over years was that distressing new community events kept occurring. We processed two new police shootings of civilians, one in which a Somali American officer killed an unarmed White woman who had called 911 because she thought she was in danger, and one in which a White officer killed an armed Black man who was running away from police officers. The community members heard the anguish that the officers felt about these shootings (most had never fired their weapon and dreaded the thought of taking someone's life). The officers came to see how generations of mistrust of law enforcement left community members feeling outraged and sometimes numb—and not at all focused (in the way the officers were) on the details of whether the shooting was legally or procedurally justified. In our conversations, the officers came to show emotion rather than only focusing on the procedural specifics of the incident, and community members became willing to listen to what had happened from the officers' perspectives. An example: The community members were upset that the police started chasing the armed man in front of his girlfriend and baby after he shot his gun into the sidewalk and someone called 911 ("The brother was standing there with his girlfriend and baby; he was not threatening them"). The officers pointed out that their colleagues were responding to a call about a shooter and would have no way to know in advance that those standing near him were related to him.

Through it all, we kept returning to the same table, not giving up on one another or our mission. Sometimes there were tears and frustrated anger, but we kept coming back to the table.

PHASE 5: A BROTHERHOOD FORMS

As the months went by, group members began to talk about their sense of friendship and even brotherhood and their pride from having difficult conversations and staying in relationship. The group sometimes laughingly recalled our "greatest hits" arguments and teased the two members who had been gladiators for their sides. When one of these two missed a meeting, group members would sometimes ask who was going to step into their combatant role! The group began to tease me about my tight control of the process— check-ins, written agendas, redirecting at times, check-outs—a control that became looser over time as the group matured.

As the climate in the group became more open and trusting, the officers increasingly shared their experiences with the human tragedies and scary situations on the job. Some recounted stories of being taunted and ridiculed on the streets because of how the public judged the actions of other officers, especially after police shootings. A community member offered this perspective: "You're being profiled. Welcome to the club." One meeting focused on supporting an officer who had come upon a horrific crime scene and was having trouble sleeping. In another meeting we supported a community member who had become unemployed and homeless and was struggling to not give up hope for personal and community change. Two officers rallied to help him get housing and a job.

One incident stands out in particular. In the middle of the night I got up from sleep to use the bathroom and heard the iPhone in my home office buzz with an incoming text. Normally I would not check texts at that hour, but that night I did. It was from one of the White officers saying that he would not be able to continue with the group because he could not handle any more intensity in his life after what had just happened during his shift. He wrote that he was searching in the snow for evidence after a drive-by shooting during which a 10-year-old girl was caught in the crossfire. What he found was her bloody tooth—she had been shot through her cheek. The street environment around him was flooded by flashing red police car lights that made it seem like he was in a Christmas horror movie as he stood there holding the bloody tooth. He thought of his own daughter who was home sleeping. He wrote that he regretted letting the group down but that he could not stay in the project and deal with the emotions involved. I texted him back with support and understanding and suggested he not make a decision right away but wait a day or two. First thing in the morning I called two community members in the group to tell them what had happened and to say that our brother officer was hurting and thinking of leaving the group. They immediately reached out to him. He decided to stay in the group, texting me that afternoon to say that he felt better and would hang in there.

Back to our meetings: As we continued to explore the bigger picture of policing and the Black community, we had the breakthrough realization that police officers and Black men are subject to similar dehumanizing stereotypes in the larger culture. In the language we developed together, both groups are seen as violent, dangerous, impulsive, uneducated, and having broken families. This insight led to conversations about how officers and Black men have become scapegoats for broader societal problems. Crime is a byproduct of neighborhoods lacking enough income, jobs, housing, health care, educational opportunities, and other resources. Police are sent in to control situations they did not create in communities that do not trust them. A sense began to emerge in our group that both sides have a common "enemy"; they are pitted against each other in a way that dehumanizes all of them.

PHASE 6: DEVELOPING OUR NARRATIVE

After we knew we had formed something solid, we decided to develop a common narrative statement to describe what we believed about the sources of mistrust between police and Black men, about what we envisioned for a better future, and about what we could do together to make a difference (see Exhibit 9.2). A key step was the decision to focus on the goal of community safety, not just better policing, because community safety is much bigger than policing. We had a consensus that there was no way to simply police communities into becoming safe to live in. A safe community, we knew, was one that fosters healthy relationships—and these relationships require an environment with opportunities to forge productive lives.

One of the community members who had experience with developing narrative statements led us through the process of writing ours. He told me afterward that some groups that are more homogeneous develop their narrative statement over several hours. Ours took months of biweekly meetings,

EXHIBIT 9.2. Minneapolis Police and Black Men Project Narrative

Abbreviated Version

Why Is There Distrust Between Black Men and Police Officers?

- There is a history of police being used to enforce and protect an unjust status quo.
- Police and Black men lack a shared understanding and relationship with each other.
- There are underlying issues (poverty, family instability, housing, education, health care, and others) that undermine the ability to build relationships for community safety.
- There are common, dehumanizing, media-driven stereotypes about each of us (both Police and Black men) that pit us against each other.

We Share These Beliefs

- That we have a common goal of community safety
- That we can't police our way out of the problem of lack of community safety
- That ongoing police training, while necessary, is not the solution
- That we each catch the blame for lack of community safety, and that we have to get closer together to address the problem and make a difference
- That people in power think they know best and share no blame for the problems facing us and the community

We Imagine a Safe Community

- Where people are in relationship with each other and have a sense of community
- Where people watch out for one another
- Where the neighborhoods are safe and clean for kids and families
- Where bad things still happen, but justice is restorative and healing and not just focused on punishment
- Where police are part of the community, trusted and honored as resources not to be feared
- Where black men can go anywhere without fear

How Do We Build a Safe Community?

- The first step is to change the story about Police and Black men. Current narratives focus either on Police Accountability Only or Personal Responsibility Only. While each of these narratives makes valid points, the upshot is finger pointing and lack of meaningful change.
- We are proposing a new narrative: Partnership for Community Safety, in which Police and Black men are allies to help the community become safe, developing closer relationships so that Black men feel safer with Police and officers' jobs are easier.
- Partnerships for community safety can also lead to joint work for systemic changes, such as initiatives for Police and community groups to work together for affordable housing so that people can feel safe and secure in their homes—and officers are not called to handle problems arising from highly stressful living situations.

partly because we had to struggle to find language that we could agree on. For example, we did not all agree on using the term *White supremacy* (to the White officers, it connoted apartheid South Africa), and yet we agreed on alternative phrases that carried similar meanings. The lesson: Go for consensus on meanings rather than specific terms. We knew we had to all stand behind every idea and word in the narrative—and the group obsessed about them. An abbreviated 1-page version of our narrative as well as the full 4-page version can be found at https://www.policeandblackmen.org.

As we worked on the narrative document, we sensed that we were breaking new ground in conversations about police and the Black community. To make a public impact, we knew we had to name and push back against two most prominent narratives and their solutions: the "just change the police" narrative (e.g., Deivanayagam et al., 2021) and the "individuals should just be more responsible" narrative (Beckett, 1999). The first comes out of the more progressive political side and the second from the more conservative side. But they each frame one-sided solutions that pit police and Black communities against each other, and neither approach alone, we believed, would lead to safer communities. We framed our narrative proposal as "Partnership for Community Safety." Safe communities are good for community members and good places for police to work and live. And that means that both the police and the community have a stake in creating the social and structural conditions for safe communities: housing security, jobs, education, health care, and other factors. The housing issue grabbed the group the most because one of our members, as mentioned, was facing housing insecurity and because the officers regularly faced messy and dangerous 911 calls over fights about who was going to stay in or leave a house. Often a man was being kicked out with nowhere to go, which in Minnesota winters can be dangerous. The officers viscerally hated removing people and making them homeless because they couldn't pay rent or had a relationship break up. "That's not why I went into policing," one officer told the group.

PHASE 7: INITIATING ACTION STEPS

When we turned our focus to what we would do together, we decided to work at three levels:

- *community conversations* to listen, to share our narrative and our story about what's possible for police and Black men to do together, and to invite community members to connect with our work;

- *police training* so that we can influence the next generation of officers; and

- *advocacy for systemic change,* with an initial focus on safe, affordable housing.

We began the community conversations after developing desired outcomes and a plan that would involve lots of group participation. The initial community gatherings were rich and impactful. They included high school students in a class sponsored by the Minneapolis Public Schools' Office of Black Male Student Achievement) and a group of men in the FATHER Project in Minneapolis. These groups talked about their fears and mistrust of the police, and then when asked to envision a safe community, they spontaneously came up with the elements of our narrative of shared partnership. We knew we were onto something.

Our next step was a meeting with the new police chief. He gave us the go-ahead to be involved in police training and embraced our idea of the police department advocating for safe housing as a public safety issue. He subsequently began that public advocacy in his role as police chief, making an explicit connection between housing security and community safety. Just as health care professionals talk about the social determinants of health, here was a police leader talking about housing as a major social determinant of community safety.

We then did our first training workshop with a new class of police cadets. We asked the same questions as in the community conversations: the sources of mistrust, participants' vision of a safe community, and how police and community members (Black men in particular) can work together to achieve safe communities for everyone. It was as potent as the community conversations, with over-the-top written evaluations from cadets. We began to talk about holding follow-up meetings with cadets after they started their field training.

Then we hit our first roadblock. The new head of cadet training decided to double down on what she considered the training basics, which did not leave room in the curriculum for our involvement. Unfortunately, the chief did not insist that we be included in the training, and the senior officer in our group did not have a good enough working relationship with the training director to get her to change her mind. This was discouraging because police training was one of the pillars of our work plan.

The second roadblock was the COVID pandemic, which shut down our community conversations. (We had a major event scheduled at a local community center the week the pandemic lockdown occurred.) We also lost our in-person meeting venues and shifted to Zoom meetings. The officers were still doing their police work in person and had to deal with daily risk of infections and medical complications, while most of the community members worked from home, and some lost jobs.

THE GEORGE FLOYD EARTHQUAKE

I clearly remember where I was sitting at my home office when one of the community members called to tell me to check out a disturbing video of a police officer ending the life of a Black man on a Minneapolis street (Eichstaedt et al., 2021). I was horrified and nauseated while watching those 7-plus minutes. I wanted to turn away, but I knew I had to watch it all because of our project. We called an emergency Zoom meeting of our group for the next day. The meeting design was basic: Let each person say what was on his heart and mind about what had happened and then discuss implications for our work. It was an agonized conversation, with tears and hot anger coming from the community members (some of whom said that George Floyd could have been them or their sons) and shock and dismay coming from the officers. There was some relief for the community members when two of the officers said plainly that Officer Chauvin had been completely out of bounds in his actions. The officers did not try to parse this incident in terms of technical rules of procedure—it was wrong. When my turn came to share, I did not maintain my typical neutrality about incidents we had discussed. I offered the thought that Chauvin kept his knee on George Floyd's neck as a way to let the distressed bystanders know that he was in charge and not them—"Don't tell me what to do. I'm the policeman." One of the officers agreed with me—he saw the same thing in Chauvin's face. Some of the officers who had worked in Chauvin's precinct in the past shared what they sensed about him—a loner with an attitude who may have become a training officer because he liked authority, and not enough other veteran officers would take on that responsibility (that was a systemic problem). They also speculated that he had been in the same precinct too long and seemed cynical and burned out years ago, something that the MPD was not good at catching and addressing.

The conversation hit rock bottom when someone noted that the two rookie trainees involved in the incident looked like two men from our cadet training class. A quick glance at that cadet roster indicated it was so. This felt like a second body blow: Two cadets with whom we discussed respect and partnership had stood by while their training officer violated the core mandate of policing to protect and serve. The officers in our group said they felt sympathy for the rookie trainees, given the authoritarian culture of the department. Their careers were likely over if they intervened and were definitely over now that they did not intervene. Some of the community members wondered what they would have done if they had been at that intersection watching the event, feeling the same bind: dive at Chauvin and be arrested for assaulting an officer, or stand and watch a brother be put to death.

The question of implications for our future work came down to a decision to keep meeting for now and sort things out later. We knew a massive storm was coming to our community—and it turns out, across the nation and the world—as outraged protestors were already taking to the streets. I can't speak for the whole group, but I felt that the action phase of our project had come to naught. What we had left—and it was meaningful—was our relationship bonds. We would go on.

Our next meetings focused on concerns about the damage to the Twin Cities community from protests that turned violent and destructive. I got a call one night from a community member who feared that one of our officers was at the Third Precinct building, which was being torched by protestors. It turned out that the officer was present and feared that his life was over. Community members of our group were on the streets as much as they could to be a calming presence, an indication that they felt like community leaders. The building that housed the FATHER Project and the Citizen Father Project was set on fire. Officers reported that they were being subjected to verbal harassment on the streets, mostly by White people as the "defund the police" movement took hold, while Black residents of communities where crime was breaking out told officers they welcomed more police presence. In our group, the emotional support flowed both ways as we witnessed Minneapolis and the MPD became poster children worldwide for racism and police brutality (Onookome-Okome et al., 2022). More than a decade of MPD work on community policing and minority police recruiting had been swept away in 7 minutes on a Minneapolis street.

Over the following months, our group began to shrink. One officer went on disability for posttraumatic stress disorder; his words: "I can't take another riot." He called me for support, and I helped him get to a therapist who might be better for him than his current one. Another officer in our group decided that he had enough of the backlash and took a job in another part of the state. There had already been attrition among the community members, with two having moved out of town, and a third took a new work position that ruled out participating in project meetings. We were down to three officers (two White and one Black) and four community members.

I wasn't sure if we had a future as the pandemic wore on, and our monthly Zoom meetings, with no action in between, seemed to be a slim thread holding us together during a time when the pandemic, MPD's defensive crouch, and community anger kept us from working on our mission in public.

PHASE 8: RECOVERY AND NEW VISIONING

Once we were able to resume in-person meetings, a recovery set in. A community member stepped up in leadership to propose a renewal of community conversations based on seeking funding support for a group of officers and Black men to travel to a museum of Black history in Montgomery, Alabama, and then raising funds to bring other groups and offer community workshops afterward. Planning for that project is underway as of this writing. An outreach from Portland, Oregon, about our work generated interest in the conversation process we had developed. Energy returned to our monthly meetings.

Although it's not clear what the project's future work will look like, one thing is clear: As the remaining Black officer put it, "We are family now." Large-scale events have set us back, but we have endured and are looking for new ways for this unlikely band of brothers to make a difference in the world.

PART **V** BECOMING AND
SUCCEEDING
AS A CITIZEN
THERAPIST

10 CASE STUDIES IN OTHER CITIZEN THERAPIST WORK

In this chapter, we describe the work of other citizen therapists. Some have published their work, which we summarize, and others have written about their projects specifically for this chapter. Echoing what we described in Chapter 1, their work goes beyond traditional outreach efforts such as public speaking, blogging, and advocating for the profession. It involves partnering with other citizens and activating the resources of ordinary people to solve problems and help one another. Professional expertise is "on tap," not "on top," and always in partnership with the life expertise of community members.

SUPPORTING GIRLS' HOLISTIC DEVELOPMENT IN SENEGAL: A GRANDMOTHER PROJECT

Note from Bill and Tai: *Here we describe the work of Judi Aubel; she is the executive director and cofounder of the Grandmother Project. This summary is based on a chapter she wrote entitled "Promoting Community-Driven Change*

https://doi.org/10.1037/0000378-011
Becoming a Citizen Therapist: Integrating Community Problem-Solving Into Your Work as a Healer, by W. J. Doherty and T. J. Mendenhall

in Family and Community Systems to Support Girls' Holistic Development in Senegal" (see Aubel, 2022).

The Grandmother Project, officially called the Grandmother Project—Change Through Culture, is situated in Southern Senegal (Aubel, 2022; Shaw et al., 2020). This region in Western Africa is considerably poor by contemporary Western standards. Poverty is rampant, and only a few communities have electricity. Families are organized in collectivist ways, with men maintaining hierarchal power over women. Boys' education is prioritized over girls', albeit all schools are both sparse and low performing. Girls rarely continue their education after reaching puberty, whereupon they are routinely betrothed in early marriages. Teen pregnancies are common, as is female genital mutilation (FGM).

When an international nonprofit organization called World Vision first asked the Grandmother Project to partner with it to strategize ways to reduce FGM in the Vélingara area of Senegal, leaders across both groups set out to explore whether what they felt as a pressure point was shared by local community members. They maintained that it was "important to foster an environment where community members are viewed as the experts of the situation" (Aubel, 2022, p. 67). They hosted numerous interviews and small-group meetings with male leaders, religious leaders, men and women, elders, health workers, and local nongovernmental organization staff. Shared sentiments revealed through these dialogues centered on wants to (a) reduce harmful traditions such as FGM while (b) improving communication between elders, parents, and children to promote positive cultural traditions. Furthermore, community members consistently identified grandmothers as key in the advancement of any intervention(s) driven by these wants, insofar as female elders are seen as primarily responsible for preserving cultural norms and because they would have the most likelihood of persuading the men who performed FGM to discontinue the practice.

As the group, now represented by both professionals and community members (men and women, adults and elders), worked together to design what would become the Girls' Holistic Development Program, they began by identifying shared objectives. Key ones were to promote positive cultural values and traditions (and discourage harmful ones), build upon existing community resources, and actively involve communication among elders, adults, and children.

From this foundation, the group advanced a series of community dialogues aimed at consensus-building for beneficent and normative change. Principal goals and desired outcomes of these dialogues included the following: (a) to increase solidarity and communication between three generations of men and women, (b) to strengthen knowledge and capacity of leaders (across three generations) to catalyze change, (c) to increase girls' self-confidence and sense of empowerment, and (d) to strengthen alliances between girls, mothers, and grandmothers.

These community dialogues purposefully engaged both professionals and lay leaders in facilitating group meetings, teaching key content, and promoting discussions about how to realize the above-described goals. The dialogues took place across a myriad of coordinated formats, including the following:

- intergenerational forums (composed of three generations of men and women together with community leaders, teachers, and health workers)

- events to honor grandmothers

- trainings for grandmother leaders in child and adolescent development and positive interpersonal communication

- trainings for teachers about positive cultural values and traditions

- workshops for grandmothers and teachers to promote better collaboration

- "under-the-tree" conversations for children, mothers, and grandmothers to strengthen communication and relationships through storytelling, games, and discussions

- all-women forums to strengthen relationships between community members and teachers and support their shared responsibility for all girls (not just their own daughters)

- all-community forums (called "Days of Dialogue and Solidarity") during which everyone discusses what they are doing and articulates future plans and actions

External evaluations (qualitative, quantitative) of this project have yielded promising results, including lower rates of FGM, less child marriage, fewer teen pregnancies, better intergenerational communication, more inclusive and gender-equitable decision making in families, and more elder and community support for girls' education. Key lessons learned through the development and implementation of the program are many (see Aubel, 2022, for a thorough discussion); they center on the importance of approaching sensitive topics with respectful and inclusive dialogue, multiple-issue (vs. single-issue) programming, engaging formal and informal leaders, and engaging multiple generations simultaneously.

Reflections from Bill and Tai: *We look forward to watching the work of the Girls' Holistic Development Program continue, evolve, and grow in scope. We see this complex combination of community dialogues as a large citizen therapist project that is truly more than the sum of its parts.*

COMMUNITY-ENGAGED RESPONSES TO THE SEPTEMBER 11TH TERRORIST ATTACKS: FROM COLLECTIVE TRAUMA TO COLLECTIVE HEALING

Note from Bill and Tai: *Here we describe the work of Jack Saul, a psychologist with an individual, couple, and family therapy practice in New York City. We wrote this overview of some of his citizen therapist work based on chapters from his book* Collective Trauma, Collective Healing: Promoting Community Resilience in the Aftermath of Disaster *(Saul, 2022).*

Works by Jack Saul and colleagues (N. Baron et al., 2003; Saul, 2000) have contributed a number of valuable insights and practical guidelines for mental health practitioners across a variety of sibling disciplines who engage with survivors of human-caused and natural disasters. Common threads through these contributions are (a) recognition of strengths and resilience within communities and (b) pairing of professional expertise with community strengths in ways that are thoughtful, culturally sensitive, and contextually appropriate.

During the weeks immediately following the attacks, Saul described himself as simultaneously a professional (a mental health provider, educator, consultant) and a community member (a resident of Lower Manhattan, a parent of two young children who were attending school near the Twin Towers). Embracing these dual identities, he and others set out to engage local parents invested in promoting the safety and well-being of their children and to support local providers working on the edge of burnout.

Beginning with a town hall meeting convened by Saul and his colleagues, parents joined together to voice and share their concerns with each other and to collectively agree upon ways to prioritize and address said concerns. Instead of waiting for overwhelmed government agencies to tackle the problems, the parents began educating themselves about air quality assessment methods and partnering with independent inspectors to test nearby schools. And instead of seeking therapy on their own (or suffering in isolation), parents began supporting each other. They did this from the clear, immediate, and shared experiences among them by nature of surviving the 9/11 attacks and from the foundations of historical experiences with trauma (because many came from diverse communities around the world experiencing civil war, political unrest, etc.). Group facilitators and professionals provided psychoeducation about common experiences related to these traumas (physical, psychological, relational), with an emphasis on self- and mutual help instead of formal treatment. Although he noted that "single-patient therapy is important to some," Saul (2022) recognized that this could not be the lead intervention in this context. Instead, "a social approach [was] essential for the wider community" (p. 79).

Along with these efforts, Saul and colleagues trained local professionals for the influx of patients seeking their help, with special attention to collegial support and self-care geared toward burnout prevention. They offered safe spaces for providers to support each other (not 1:1 therapy with therapists). They imparted content knowledge (e.g., regarding clinical care for trauma survivors during early and later time periods postdisaster), with careful consideration for how to coordinate and triage services in culturally sensitive ways.

As the weeks following the 9/11 attacks turned into months, these and related efforts continued and evolved. Primary needs identified by community members (professional and lay) included ongoing attention to environmental safety, monitoring and responding to children's and adults' psychological functioning, sustaining social support and cohesion, and making clear and useful information available about all of these foci. Within local schools, parents and teachers worked together to clean up neighborhoods and school facilities, to maintain supportive spaces to learn about common trauma sequelae (e.g., regressive behaviors in children over long-term recovery processes), and to offer and receive peer support (supplemented by professional psychoeducation and related resources). They advocated for respite and vacation time for teachers' self-care and well-being. They also created short and long educational and documentary videos to serve as tools for ongoing education and project development. Offshoot initiatives from these larger efforts have advanced similar pursuits: for example, a local neighborhood project working to advocate for affordable housing, a local school project using samba (music, dancing) as a supportive outlet for youth, a group of journalists focused on supporting each other and their broader profession as an often high-risk group, a group of actors using theater to share broadly felt experiences of trauma.

Outcome data yielded by the multiple community projects described above—and over their multiple years of programming—are myriad. In addition to results already described (e.g., neighborhood cleanups, teachers' time off, clinicians' preparedness, normalization of and support for self-care), formally and informally tracked results coalesced across the following themes: (a) enhanced social connectedness; (b) opportunities for shared storytelling, validation, and support; (c) collective healing rituals; and (d) a renewed sense of hope. These outcomes pertained to lay community members and professionals alike.

Reflections from Bill and Tai: *The work described here represents several key principles of citizen health care. It is clear that Saul (2022) immediately recognized two broad and essential sources of expertise in responding to the tragedies of the 9/11 terror attacks. The first is professional; he identified himself as a mental health care provider and as an educator and expert in the interdisciplinary field of trauma recovery. He is clear, too, throughout his narrative about the ways that his and his colleagues' scientific and clinical expertise is informative to both early- and long-term community programming. The second broad and essential source of expertise that Saul (2022) recognized is community—that is, that the greatest untapped resource for improving health and social well-being is the lived experience of the individuals, families, and larger groups that we offer care to. Explicitly, he maintains that (a) "communities have the capacity to heal themselves" and that (b) "the greatest resources for recovery are the community members, themselves" (p. 122).*

EMPOWERING MEN TO RECOVER FROM DEPRESSION: THE FACE IT FOUNDATION

MARK MEIER

Note from Bill and Tai: *Mark Meier is a colleague in the Twin Cities who has done noteworthy citizen therapist work with men dealing with depression. He wrote the following in response to our invitation to share his journey with the Face It Foundation.*

I (Mark) earned my master's of social work in 1994 and my licensed independent clinical social worker designation in 1998, and in 2001 found myself the administrator of a large dialysis clinic in Minneapolis. I was married, had three amazing children, owned a house and a nice car, was saving for college for my children and my own retirement, was advancing in my career, had friends, and was active in my community. By all outward measures, my life was heading in the "right" directions. However, hidden deep under the layers of my successes were the pains of depression, anxiety, past traumas, and an unhealthy relationship with alcohol. I battled a constant sense of inadequacy; felt like a failure; found no joy in anything; and presumed that my wife, children, colleagues, friends, and the world in general would be better off without me.

By the end of 2002, I had made a suicide attempt, dealt with an acute psychiatric hospitalization, completed an intensive outpatient mental health program, started taking medication for my depression and anxiety, was attending a 12-step program, and had started and stopped outpatient individual psychotherapy a couple of times. In the span of little over 1 year, I had gone from a mental health professional to a consumer of multiple mental health services, and it was during this time that I began to take note of the missing piece that no mental health professional or program could provide me with: friendship. Sure, I had friends, in fact lots of them, but very few felt accessible to me to truly share what I had been through. And those who did care deeply about me had never experienced any of the traumas and pain I had endured. I felt intolerably lonely.

I was eager to begin meeting other men like me, to share my story and to hear theirs, to find a bond with others who were trying to raise their children, grow their career, be a good husband, and learn from the experiences of life with depression, anxiety, and posttraumatic stress disorder. I asked my psychiatrist where I could find these men, how I could begin to build friendships with them, and how I could learn from them. The blank stare and silence that met my request spoke volumes. My psychiatrist cared for other patients like me, but of course he couldn't introduce me to them or connect us in any way. I asked, "Surely you have a support group for men like me?" Again, nothing. My worst fear was confirmed: I was an ugly anomaly who would have to go through life holding all my secrets inside.

Fast forward a few years, and I find myself teaching a mood disorders seminar in a graduate school of social work. One of the assignments I created for my students was to identify, read, and discuss the merits of a self-help book focused on depression. The point of this exercise was to help trainees look beyond the usual interventions of cognitive behavior therapy, dialectical behavior therapy, interpersonal therapy, and so on and encourage them to see ways in which clients can help themselves to grow. In one section of the class, our conversation turned to clients using self-help, but several students stated they didn't see the value of it. They believed that the only real path to recovery from a mood disorder was 1:1 therapy. As this conversation continued, I introduced the concept of peer support; this notion was also met with skepticism. Although I respected my students' opinions, I took note and began to wonder if there were additional biases against the use of peer support or self-help in the minds of other mental health professionals.

During the time I was teaching in the school of social work, I was running my own consulting business to bring awareness and focused interventions to the management of chronic diseases (specifically, diabetes and kidney disease) for patients who also suffered from mood and anxiety disorders. This work put me in front of hundreds of mental health professionals across the United States. I started speaking more about the role of peer support. I gave more than 400 talks and trainings, but only in very few instances was my advocacy for peer support embraced. As an example: At a large conference focused on suicide prevention, I presented my ideas as a keynote speaker. Audience evaluations about the content of my talk were remarkably critical. One comment that really stuck with me, for example, was a responder who challenged the event organizers with a question to the effect of "How could someone with dangerous ideas about using peer support in place of therapy be allowed to present at a conference on suicide prevention?"

In a training that I delivered to a group of nephrologists at an annual chronic kidney disease summit, I spoke about the impact of mood disorders on kidney disease. I also spoke openly—for the first time—about my own struggles with depression. What struck me at this event wasn't the criticism about peer support as topic but rather a physician who approached me to quietly share his own struggles with depression. He described how he longed to be able to speak openly with his colleagues but feared for his professional image and reputation. The irony of this was that I had met hundreds of health care professionals who had shared with me similar personal struggles, and all felt they had to live quietly with their pain and shame.

In 2009, I founded the Face It Foundation. I had reached a breaking point of sorts. I was weary of my own sense of isolation, as a man and as a health provider. I was weary of hearing so many professionals' disparaging public remarks about peer support while privately sharing with me their hardships with depression and their shame about getting help.

The mission of Face It reads: "Leveraging the power of peer support, Face It works with men to recover from depression and prevent suicide." Today, our foundation serves more than 200 men with multiple services. Our primary approach to helping men is through peer-led support.

The first Face It group was launched in December 2011 with eight men. As was intended from the outset, the group was solely a place to share experiences with depression (e.g., loneliness, fear, shame, abandonment), relationship difficulties (e.g., with spouse, partner, children, parents, siblings, colleagues), behavioral challenges (e.g., violence, anger, fights), addictions (e.g., alcohol and other substances, gambling, pornography, sex), and successes and failures with treatment (e.g., medications, talk therapies). This model (8–10 men plus facilitators) has endured as an effective standard for how ensuing groups have formed and evolved.

Prior to anyone joining a group, I meet individual members personally so as to have a chance to get to know them better. During this initial meeting, I do not make any diagnostic assessments. I use the time to share stories about recovery, learn what the individual is looking for, and explain the ways in which our groups function. Many men who come through our doors are looking for connection to others, along with a place to talk about what they have gone through in their lives.

My estimate is that 80% of Face It participants have participated in some type of therapy before and therein have been formally diagnosed with depression, an anxiety disorder, a substance use issue, or bipolar disorder. Many I have met have stories of being physically or sexually abused as a child, with many revealing to us, for the first time, this history. Many of the men are divorced or in partnerships they describe as "empty," "loveless," or "convenient" or any variety of other terms that connote a lack of intimacy. Many who have adult children have strained relationships with them or are estranged altogether. Most of our guys have attempted suicide, and some continue to live with ongoing suicidal ideation. I estimate that 90% of them carry a deep sense of shame about these things and have very little sense of self. The men who come to Face It, by and large, are gainfully employed or retired. We have served physicians, attorneys; CEOs; police officers, fire-fighters, and emergency medical technicians; military; blue-collar workers; and just about any other type of profession you might think of. The men we serve are often the ones whom society would perceive as having it all together.

Two men (usually laypersons) facilitate most groups. Having two men allows for the absence of one guy when things come up, and it provides the facilitators with a sense of support. The men who facilitate our groups have been in a Face It group themselves; over time they found themselves doing better and then stepped up to lead a group. We support our facilitators with 1- to 2-hour trainings six times a year. These trainings are not mandatory, but they are very well-attended. I also speak with most facilitators one or two times a month. Prior to taking on a group, I meet with the facilitators two or three times to talk about appropriate boundaries, communication strategies, how to handle challenging situations, and what to do if someone talks about being suicidal. I help them, too, to craft strategies for the first few meetings.

Impact of the Peers

As noted above, by wearing my mental health professional "hat," I am able to provide some guidance and oversight to the peer group leaders. Our facilitators, however, are responsible for what takes place in their individual groups. Face It doesn't have formal steps to rely on or guide us, and we don't have a prescribed (or proscribed) format for the meetings. In fact, though many

12-step groups discourage cross-talk, at Face It we promote and encourage interaction, feedback, and dialogue. Peers also decide on ground rules for their specific group, and they establish expectations around attendance and participation.

There are many ways in which the peer model plays out within our groups and impacts the well-being of members. A conspicuous example is that the peer facilitators are members of the group, just like any of the members—from the guy who has been in group for months to the one who just started. In my observation and experience, men are more likely to open up about their struggles when they perceive similarities with those they are sharing with. I have heard on many occasions from men that they don't trust therapists because they know nothing about them (reciprocally) and have no sense about whether or not the therapist even understands what they are dealing with. In a peer model, there is a flat hierarchy, and facilitators use group time for their own benefit like everyone else.

Our peer groups include a great deal of storytelling. When men are given time and space to fully develop a narrative around their experiences with depression, both from a mood experience and from a behavioral or life experience, a tremendous amount of information is shared. What has been well-documented by the men of Face It is that they learn a lot about themselves and their own coping mechanisms when listening to the experiences of others. Many men come to a peer group with difficulties opening up about their experiences, but by being given the latitude to be present and just listen (unlike 1:1 therapy where a client is expected to actively engage), they are able to integrate new ideas and approaches helpful in their own recovery process.

Perhaps the most important aspect of the peer group is the relationships and friendships that are developed outside of the actual group. Face It has fostered hundreds of new friendships that in turn have provided men with not only a resource in the face of an acute issue but also the ongoing and needed support to encourage and promote recovery. The concept of "accountability" is widespread among the men, and most would say that it is based on the sense of responsibility one feels toward a friend. These men have talked about making changes in their lives because they raised an issue in a group and the other men encouraged or even pushed them to become healthier. This initial reason for change often leads to a deeper understanding of oneself, and many men continue to grow because they come to realize the benefits of making changes for their own well-being. This pattern, as I see it, is driven in large part initially by the sense of responsibility to others in the group.

Outside of the peer groups, the 28 men who facilitate our groups also support one another. Face It creates monthly opportunities for facilitators to gather and talk about their experiences and their own needs that come about from leading groups. Many of our facilitators initially have a difficult time not feeling responsible for the men in their group, for example, and through conversations and modeling they begin to see what they can influence and what is beyond their control.

Impact on Me

As a mental health professional, I still believe in the power of psychotherapy, but my beliefs have evolved over time in that I see greater opportunities for clinicians who provide therapies such as eye movement desensitization and reprocessing, accelerated resolution therapy, brainspotting, and other trauma-based approaches. My sense of traditional talk therapy, unless guided by skilled clinicians, is that a peer group is equally—if not more—effective. And certainly, even in the case of a skilled clinician providing a modality such as cognitive behavior therapy, a peer group enhances the experience and provides the individual who is suffering with the opportunity to develop an ongoing relationship with a peer. (My bias, based on 30-plus years of experience, is that far too many clinicians who claim expertise in certain therapies are not as competent as they perceive.)

When I first launched Face It, I was nervous about putting peers in charge of groups, but I quickly witnessed and experienced (using my peer experiences way more than my clinical skills) just how much faster men gravitated to my story of depression, suicidality, and recovery than they did to any clinical information I tried to relate. This connection, in turn, gave permission to the men in our groups to share their own stories, to ask their own questions about recovery, and to challenge their own beliefs and ideas about what they were experiencing. And most important, these conversations were (are) ongoing and could occur 1, 2, 3, or more days a week, not just during the 50 minutes they had scheduled for a therapy visit.

One of the truest testaments to the power of peer support has been in our ability to prevent suicides. Face It works with a high percentage of men who represent one of the highest risk categories for suicide (middle-aged White males), and in 14-plus years we have lost only one man who was actively engaged in a Face It group. I have hundreds of examples of men having suicidal thoughts who have reached out to others in their group at all hours (day or night) and on all days of the week looking for help. The support and guidance provided by these peers toward their friend who was suicidal has been pivotal and—literally—lifesaving!

Reflections from Bill and Tai: *What is immediately clear to us in Mark's narrative is that the Face It Foundation was founded on a shared pressure point defined by the pain, stigma, shame, and isolation that many men who are living with depression and other mental health struggles feel. Mark's lived experience with these struggles reflected both sides of the professional and personal equation, as a provider and as a consumer of conventional services. Resistance from the professional community (skepticism about the value of peer support) and the felt ineffectiveness of top-down-only services from the lay community further fueled Mark's desire to do something different. Citizen health care is founded on the principle that the greatest untapped resource for improving health is the knowledge, wisdom, and energy of individuals, families, and communities who face challenging health issues in their everyday lives. Men who are struggling in the manner that Mark describes maintain insider perspectives about their journeys in pain, healing, and growth that cannot be understood by reading a textbook. Face It facilitates flat-hierarchy conversations, sharing, accountability, and support. Mark helps to prepare and support facilitators in their work (professional expertise "on tap," not "on top"), with the key being that these lay facilitators have "been there, done that." They function in the same manner as other group participants: as men who are supporting and receiving support from other men (lived community experience). The concern that Face It participants have for each other—paired with the outward-facing visibility of the foundation's message though its literature, website, and related community efforts—is a clear testament to the power of citizen therapist work to tackle a serious social problem.*

WORKING WITH COMMUNITIES TO PROMOTE THE WELLNESS OF BLACK FAMILIES IN MIAMI: THE CRECER LAB

MARISOL L. MEYER, ALEXIS R. FRANKLIN, CEEWIN N. LOUDER, JOELLE DORSETT, MARIE BOURSIQUOT WHITE, AND GUERDA NICOLAS

Note from Bill and Tai: *Marisol Meyer is a doctoral candidate in counseling psychology at the University of Miami in the School of Education and Human Development. She responded to an invitation that we sent to her program asking for examples of current efforts in citizen therapy projects. We then invited her and her colleagues to contribute a write-up describing their efforts in the CRECER lab.*

Derived from the Spanish word *crecer,* meaning "to grow," the Challenging Racism and Empowering Communities through Ethnocultural Research (CRECER) team is a community-based participatory research initiative based in South Florida at the University of Miami. Dr. Guerda Nicolas has led the lab for more than 13 years in tandem with doctoral, master's, and undergraduate students who are committed to social-justice–oriented academic research and community programming centering ethnic minorities and immigrant populations. Our overarching mission is to encourage community empowerment through the development of sustainable community programs for youth, families, and organizations that promote psychological and community well-being. This is achieved through community partnerships that center community strengths.

CRECER and Community Programming

CRECER's engagement centers the culturally diverse neighborhoods of the West Grove and Overtown, whose residents typically identify as African American, Bahamian, Haitian, and Jamaican. These historically Black neighborhoods are rich in culture and connectedness, though they are experiencing rapid gentrification. Community leaders have expressed that stressors related to gentrification and other forms of systemic racism more broadly have had palpable impacts on the mental health of community members. The identification of these stressors is not done casually, nor is it driven by researchers. Indeed, CRECER members and community leaders cohost an annual community engagement event. This Day of Dialogue provides community organizations with the opportunity to come together to both identify and take action to address the needs of the community. Themes for previous Days of Dialogue include Blacks in Miami, American Indians and education, well-being & self-love, race relations, and women's wellness. Through these dialogues, sustainable intervention programs for youth, families, and the surrounding community have been developed and implemented based on the needs identified by the people within the community. One of the most sustainable and generative programs is called Kulula.

The Kulula Project

The need for Kulula was presented by community members at the 2009 Day of Dialogue themed "Addressing the Needs of Blacks in Miami." Families noted that available after-school programs did not celebrate Black culture. After having multiple conversations with community leaders, both CRECER members and community partners agreed that rather than targeting a "problem," a program would be designed from a strengths-based approach to enhance the psychological well-being of Black youth. The need for this program was evident through anecdotal information shared by community leaders and in extant literature; Black youth experience substantial increases in general well-being by participating in after-school programs but participate in such programs at lower rates than do non-Black peers (Fredricks & Simpkins, 2012; Woodland, 2008).

However, we were stuck with one question: How can we create an after-school program focusing on racial–ethnic identity development that Black youth will actually find engaging? The CRECER team and leaders at the community center in which the project would be housed initially formed an adolescent advisory board to collaborate in an effort to understand what issues were important to adolescents and the best ways to address them. Board members consisted of local high school students demonstrating interest in leadership and community empowerment and who had previously engaged in a pilot version of Kulula. After combining the insight from the board with the current literature, the CRECER team created the first version of the currently used curriculum. However, when we presented this to the advisory board, they hated it! We were told that the topics were boring, the language was hard to understand, and it felt unrelatable. This feedback was crucial for entering an iterative process to finalize a curriculum that the adolescent advisory board found culturally relevant. After 5 years of quarterly action-and-planning meetings, the board and researchers were able to identify a beloved draft of the curriculum. To ensure that the curriculum remains acceptable, our team and Kulula coordinators continue to gather feedback from past and current participants to assess and improve the program.

Key Activities of the Kulula Project

The key activities of Kulula consist of guided discussions led by mentors, developmentally appropriate activities (e.g., worksheets, crafts, journaling), community celebrations, and a capstone civic engagement project. All program activities were developed through collaborative and continuous reflection processes between professional and community partners. Indeed, one way we make our values of collaborative and equitable partnership actionable is via a long-term commitment in which we meet with community partners and members multiple times throughout each year to listen to their thoughts and suggestions.

Each year begins with scheduling at least two meetings with our community partners with the central tasks of identifying both strengths and improvement areas for program implementation. In between these two annual meetings, we cohost celebratory events (i.e., Kwanzaa, Black History Month) that are open to community members regardless of participation in CRECER interventions. Indeed, community is a unit of identity, and we value the voices and participation of community members regardless of the extent of their involvement with CRECER.

A central component of program participation is the creation of a civic engagement project designed to teach youth that they have agency in their community. This project is entirely directed by the youth, who are asked to identify things in their community that they love but would like to improve. In 2021, program activities were tailored to focus on environmentalism, reflecting an increase of community conversations surrounding climate change and climate gentrification in Miami. By tailoring program activities to the implicitly and explicitly identified interests of our community partners, Kulula allowed for an emphasis on the local relevance of systemic problems.

Collaborative Assessment of the Kulula Project's Impact

Before, during, and after the implementation of a program with community partners, the CRECER lab and community partners ground the work in culturally responsive theory of change and logic models (Meyer et al., 2021). The cocreation of these models with community leaders emphasizes community voice in identification of long-term and short-term goals for programs, identification of community resources to create change, collaboration regarding how to conceptualize and recognize desired change, and dynamic and collaborative redesign of program elements informed by community feedback.

The CRECER lab and community partners have approached evaluation of the program's flexibly; the research design is always guided by immediate community needs. Although it is typically recommended that the community take part in data collection, analysis, and dissemination, our community partners expressed a preference that CRECER researchers manage these tasks. Community partners would frequently indicate that leaders and members in the community were often overwhelmed and overworked, which resulted in a limited capacity to participate in all dimensions of the research. Instead, community leaders demonstrated interest and capacity to engage in discussions related to research design and data interpretation as well as review material before its dissemination by CRECER researchers.

Assessment typically includes administration of quantitative measures and formal focus groups. Although we value both informal and formal interactions with community members, meetings are held with community leaders who have more frequent and direct contact with community members in an effort to interpret the data. The following anecdote exemplifies the value added by collaboratively interpreting data with community leaders. The Multigroup Ethnic Identity Measure (MEIM; Phinney, 1992) is a tool used to assess the impact(s) of Kulula on youth's ethnic–racial identity development. The use of this measure was at the request of community leaders interested in quantitative assessment. During data cleaning procedures, a graduate student recognized a "negative" shift in ethnic–racial identity development and assumed it to be cause for concern. However, during a formal meeting, community leaders identified that a negative trend in postintervention scores was actually a reflection of youth being exposed to discussions of race and racism for the first time. Most youth in the Kulula project spend a majority of their time in systems that undermine their ethnic–racial identity. A youth who scored high on the MEIM during the preintervention assessment may have learned the words *race* and *ethnicity* when engaging in Kulula programming. Incorporating community partners in data interpretation allowed for a reconceptualization of indicators of successful engagement with the project and further evaluation of initiatives.

Lessons Learned and Next Steps

This report has thus far been written by CRECER members consisting of cisgender women of color from various socioeconomic backgrounds. However, the lead author of this piece has written the current section. I (Marisol) am a White-presenting Cuban-American cisgender woman. I am also a graduate student at the University of Miami about to complete my doctorate in counseling psychology and have been involved with the CRECER lab for 4 years. While I have learned a great deal during my time in the lab, all my experiences are unified in that they contributed to my understanding of, and belief in, cultural humility (Tervalon & Murray-Garcia, 1998). To practice cultural humility, I strive to primarily listen and speak only when I can feel confident that my voice will not silence anyone else's. I believe not only in listening to, but hearing, our community partners. This has been a catalyst for partnership efforts inspiring change.

Similarly, community partners have shared that the experience of being heard and responded to has inspired optimism and development of leadership skills in community members with whom we work closely. I am grateful for the parallel process in which I have grown alongside the community members who have forever informed my position that mental health cannot exist without community. However, these reflections are my own. To broaden the reader's understanding of the cascading impacts that CRECER has had on more than a decade's worth of academics and community members, the following provides broader reflections on lessons learned and next steps.

All CRECER members agree on one critical lesson: relationships matter. To exemplify this point, we'd like to bring the reader back to the first Day of Dialogue. Community members and community stakeholders did not initially receive the theme "Addressing the Needs of Blacks in Miami" very well. Having recently relocated from the northeastern United States, Dr. Nicolas was perplexed as she had found this form of community action to be typically embraced. It was through many patient and uncomfortable conversations with community members that she grasped the insidious cultural forces at play. The multicultural metropolis of Miami is still a city in the South. Segregation offers tourists a manufactured experience with Caribbean cultural practices, while structural and economic forces marginalize many of those with the most authentic ties to these heritages.

These conversations highlighted that families had survived for generations by not ruffling feathers. Why would a community that found a tried-and-true way to survive for so long trust a new-in-town, hot-shot academic? She was not the first person from a university promising change. And trust takes time to develop. Yet a community leader saw promise in Dr. Nicolas's strategy for advocating with this community to work toward solving a myriad of pressure points: Mrs. Thelma Gibson.

Mrs. Gibson and her family played a significant role in shaping Miami for generations. She was committed to uplifting Black communities in South Florida through a tremendous amount of nonprofit work, advocacy, and political involvement (The HistoryMakers, 2006). When Mrs. Gibson championed the 2009 Day of Dialogue theme, community members were willing to give this sort of work a chance. The Kulula project was integrated into the Thelma Gibson Health Initiative, an organization that the community members trusted. As Dr. Nicolas and Mrs. Gibson continued to develop both the program and their relationship, they agreed to apply for a grant together. At an open hearing for the community about grant proposals, Mrs. Gibson's arrival prompted applause. The board chairman even asked all attendees to stand as she entered. Without Dr. Nicolas' and Mrs. Gibson's relationship, Kulula may never have come to fruition. In community work, relationships with community members, leaders, and stakeholders are paramount.

As gentrification worsens for Black families in South Florida, the nature of our community work has shifted to identifying ways in which to keep the community united as geography threatens the bonds they have developed as neighbors. This brings us to a similarly salient lesson learned: Collaborative work must be grounded in the recognition that the issues many Black families face are systemic, not individual. This can be difficult to grapple with, as systemic change takes considerable time and commitment. Although we should not undermine the importance of individual changes experienced by Kulula participants, we must recognize that racial inequities continue to thrive and will continue to undermine the wellness of Black families so long as they exist. A study initiated by Miami–Dade County Mayor Daniella Levine Cava, for example, found that Black residents of Miami-Dade County still feel unwelcome, unsafe, and without access to opportunities to improve their socioeconomic position (Miami-Dade County, 2021).

Why do community work if it can be so difficult? Why commit to change if you cannot be sure you will be able to see the transformation in your lifetime? Because relationships matter. As psychologists, budding psychologists, and individuals just dipping their toes into the field of psychology, members of the CRECER lab work with communities because few other types of professional work allow one to feel one's humanity so deeply. Of course, as researchers, we engage in intellectual pursuits, we collect data, and we publish manuscripts. But as CRECER team members collaborating with communities, we attend Kwanzaa celebrations, high school graduations, talent shows, protests, and funerals. We have danced together, fought together, and cried together, and we will continue to do so. Going forward, we cannot tell you the specific projects that we will undertake, but we can tell you it will be with the community members and leaders of the historically Black neighborhoods in South Florida. Further information about the CRECER lab can be found at https://sites.education.miami.edu/crecer.

Reflections from Bill and Tai: *We resonate with this project in part because we are also situated in a large university. Outreach and service efforts by academy experts are generally advanced in a top-down manner (e.g., a professor studying social–emotional learning delivers a lecture to a local school board, a physician consults with a community health clinic's staff about a new treatment-standard). And though this type of work is laudable in its own right for specific pursuits, it often falls short in allaying more complex community struggles and pressure points. From the outset of their work, CRECER professionals were clearly aware of this tendency (i.e., powerful professionals "fixing" less powerful community members) and resistant to its natural draw. As they partner with the West Grove and Overtown neighborhoods of Miami, they embody the wisdom that the greatest untapped resource in the work they are doing is within these neighborhoods (not in the academy). Their professional expertise and power is an essential part of the equations that they are collaboratively solving (e.g., via entry into and influence over conversations about, and policy changes in, curricula for after-school programming), but revisions to programmatic content, delivery methods, and data interpretation are informed and led by community members.*

It is important to note, too, that within this larger frame of "community members," it is Kulula's youth who are the most active. This is appropriate because the work's vision is about improving the lives of this community's youth. This shared ownership and cooperative work is sustained through Kulula's local community to retrieve its own historical and cultural traditions. The community is doing this through a myriad of celebrations, rituals, dance, and community conversations—all of which center on a foundation of shared history as African Americans, Bahamians, Haitians, and Jamaicans living in the West Grove and Overtown neighborhoods for several generations. We are excited to learn more about the future of this important work.

TAKING CARE OF PEOPLE WHO MAKE PEOPLE: THE HONEY. FOR MOMS PROJECT

BROOKE MILLER

Note from Bill and Tai: *Brooke Miller is a colleague in Michigan who has done innovative citizen therapist work with mothers who are navigating a host of challenges related to this complex life transition. She wrote the following in response to our invitation to share her journey with the organization called Honey. for Moms.*

I developed Honey. for Moms (Honey, for short) to elevate how maternal mental health support is defined, accessed, and utilized by humans who identify as mothers. My foundational belief is that the maternal instinct is the most powerful voice in existence, though the layers and complexities of life, society, and history have led to a dimming of that voice, and the consequences are profound. My startup goal was not for Honey and my team to simply author academic papers or guide university studies but rather to connect with mothers, as mothers, as a way to heal from the collective trauma of motherhood.

The Honey. for Moms Story

A former full-time nanny, I shifted to work as a licensed psychotherapist in 2007. When I became a mother in 2012, everything changed. What began as "baby blues"—an expression for the physical and emotional adjustment that mirrors symptoms of depression and anxiety for 1 to 2 weeks (something that up to 80% of new mothers experience)—turned into an indefatigable and at times even angry response to the lack of direct and indirect support that mothers are provided in our society.

In 2014, from a 500-square-foot rented room in the back of a chiropractor's office, I started Honey, drawing on my passion for mental health access and the power of group support. I took to social media to let local moms know there was a space for them to "gather, connect, breathe, and grow." The offering menu included moms' groups, workshops, and yoga. It quickly grew. Within a year, Honey became the 4,500-square-foot wellness center she is today, adding therapy, classes, a coworking lounge, and on-site child-care to the roster of offerings.

When the COVID-19 pandemic began shutting down many other organizations, Honey maintained its mission and roots (mental health services and community support). I launched Honey Online, which was a simple Facebook group with daily classes offered virtually, bookended by a daily sing-along for kids and families in the morning, story time offered by my own daughters, and group support every evening. Honey was written up by *The New York Times* in recognition for our pivot online (see https://www.nytimes.com/2020/06/26/business/pandemic-honey-space-online.html), and our community was more connected than ever. In May 2022, Honey's physical space reopened. Psychiatry services were added, alongside a free formula library (which was born from the formula crisis in the United States during the summer of 2022 and remains a steady offering to this day).

Current Program Content and Processes

Honey. for Moms includes formal services (vertical) offered by professionals to mothers seeking care and community support (horizontal) between mothers supporting each other. As they walk through the door, moms enter the Honey space. Curated to encourage safety, rest, and calm, the environment, adorned with candles and intentional lighting, has a completely different feel from a traditional mental health office. A custom mural *I am Honey* graces the wall with a pictorial narrative of motherhood stories including pregnancy, loss, motherhood, breastfeeding, bottle-feeding, and pumping, with C-section scars, authentic body shapes, and beautiful exhaustion illuminated in the work. Honey's aforementioned free formula library is offered to moms who need it. A library of books is available to borrow from, an infant scale and feeding chair are available, and the coffee and tea are always hot. On a wall between therapy offices is a custom experiential piece of art by HoneyMama and artist Holliday Martindale called *Noam's Om*. This space invites participation by moms to honor miscarriages and infant losses.

Honey holds a space for mothers to connect with others who are moving through the same chapter of motherhood as they are, from their first moment forward. All group leaders (professional and community) are trained in a narrative method that I call "The Honey Method"; this includes information about perinatal mental health, empathy development, and effective and evidence-based ways to facilitate group processes that feel safe and welcoming. Groups are separated by stages of motherhood, such as miscarriage and motherhood (for moms who are moving through loss while mothering), pregnancy, newborn, next born, moms of toddlers, and working moms. Other more specific groups, including though not limited to moms of children with complex medical diagnosis, LGBTQI mamas, and HoneyforDads, are on the schedule. Participants register for a 6-week series and begin with an offering of coffee or tea and a brief tour. There is stroller and car seat parking. Group guidelines include the welcoming of babies who are crying, sleeping, rocking, or feeding and for mothers to feel safe in their authentic feelings at any given moment. Group members gather on the floor with floor chairs, blankets, and pillows, and babies are in arms or cozy in front of mama. Babies are also welcome to be left with another caregiver while mama joins the group alone if that's best for her mental health. Support services centered on breast- and bottle-feeding are also available. Other people connected to moms (partners, grandparents, older siblings of new babies, etc.) are served through a combination of referrals and workshops, as well.

Online, Honey moms support each other through Facebook with approximately 1,000 active users in a private group and 7,000 followers on a public social media page. Though other staff and I curate the site to ensure that accurate information is presented, the majority of the site's work is carried out by moms connecting with other moms. They share stories and offer support through the lived experience and wisdom of maternal parenthood, from empathic narratives to simply saying "twinkle fingers" (an argot—or "honey-ism"—that says, "I get you," "I hear you," and "You are not alone").

Impact and Follow-Up

The impact of Honey is both subtle and internal for each participant and macro for the community as a whole. "Our Honey. for Moms new mama group alumni are off to kindergarten this fall!" reads a post on social media in August 2022, with a photo attached of moms and babies with Honey as the background and comments with shared photos of 5- and 6-year-olds who spent time at Honey as infants. An office wall is graced with notes, cards, and messages to Honey and her team expressing how being part of Honey changed their life, helped them be a better mother and person, and endless additional sentiments that can't help but draw an observer in to recognize how Honey is making her way into the cells of everyone who walks through her door.

Past and current HoneyMamas who participate in our private Facebook group that I manage and support, called the HoneyMama Hive, make dozens of daily posts. In addition to our current group members, there are hundreds of additional requests to join from those who have heard about Honey.

To hold the space with intention and commitment, only those who have been to Honey or participated virtually are added; this ensures that they have learned Honey's language and guidelines and are prepared to share a respectful and loving space that feels different from many other online spaces.

Beyond the personal testimonials, Honey is considering the impact of our methods and approaches to see if they are confirmed as evidence-based. For now, though, I am satisfied with the pure and consistent feedback of how deeply Honey is impacting the lives of those I am lucky enough to work with.

Next Steps

As my own motherhood has shifted from the opening of Honey (from a 2-year-old and an infant to—now—11- and 8-year-old daughters), I am called to show up and take up space as a different mother and person than I was on Honey's opening day. I originally managed the front desk, cleaning, scheduling, and group leadership in the early days, all tasks that are now held with grace by team members, giving me space for innovating and planting elsewhere in order to bring Honey's impact deeper into the world.

Honey has been asked a multitude of times over the years to franchise the concept or grow into more locations, but I have held the boundary. Being the daughter of a franchisor, I know what life I want and what kind of organization I want to lead. Franchising means ownership of the way—and though there is certainly pride and creative ownership of the process of holding the space in the HoneyWay, it is simply too impactful to contain to one space in Michigan. The impact of certain pieces of the Honey process, particularly the HoneyMethod group leadership training, is something I see as vast and reaching. Thus, having been asked by corporate environments, small businesses, religious organizations, and small groups alike to train them to offer programs for moms and parents on-site and online in their own communities, my lead team and I are considering offering the HoneyMethod to far-reaching places (but not as franchises), making certain that the empathy-based and trauma-driven model of support and collaborative care is understood, leading to a valiant expansion of our mission: To take care of the people who make, raise, nourish and grieve the people . . . and give the world the tools to do the same.

Reflections from Bill and Tai: *Brooke Miller's story shows how a citizen therapist can leverage a personal pressure point for the public good. She recognized early on that a deep response to the challenges that new mothers face would require a combination of personal and professional expertise. As she and other team leaders work on pragmatic, focused, and specific projects (classes, support groups, etc.) in response to the evolving needs of the Michigan communities within which Honey resides, they are sustained by a big, bold mission to destigmatize postpartum depression, to normalize struggles common to mothering, and to support and empower people who make people. Current media engagement and new and evolving efforts to extend Honey's reach suggest strongly that it is succeeding.*

CONCLUDING COMMENT

We are excited to see the impressive work of other citizen therapists. We hope that many iterations of this chapter can be written with new examples. We look forward to learning how therapists have engaged community members in the creation of something novel, innovative, and inspiring.

11

MAINTAINING CITIZEN HEALTH CARE PROJECTS OVER TIME

The projects described in this text tried to rally communities and professionals together around pressure points that everyone involved sees as important. So far, we have focused primarily on the startup and action phases of the work. In this chapter, we describe strategies for maintaining projects over time.

STRATEGIES FOR PROJECT SUSTAINABILITY

Though not all citizen therapist projects require a long-term focus, those that do aim for longevity require special strategies. Exhibit 11.1 outlines the strategies that we've employed to keep citizen health care projects going over time.

Involve Everyone to Identify and Articulate Pressure Points

Citizen health care projects seek to involve everyone from professionals and administrators to lay community members in identifying and articulating something that is important all-around. Recall, for example, how everyone

https://doi.org/10.1037/0000378-012
Becoming a Citizen Therapist: Integrating Community Problem-Solving Into Your Work as a Healer, by W. J. Doherty and T. J. Mendenhall

EXHIBIT 11.1. Strategies for Sustaining Projects Over Time

- Involve everyone in identifying and articulating pressure points.
- Secure institutional buy-in.
- Be careful about external funding, especially at the outset.
- Aim for transformed civic identities.
- Identify leaders and then more leaders.
- Be patient with program development.
- Be careful (always!) about the pull of the traditional provider–consumer model.
- Create ways to fold new learnings back into the community.
- Forge a sense of larger purpose.
- Obsess about effective group process.

in the Students Against Nicotine and Tobacco Addiction (SANTA) Project (see Chapter 3, this book) agreed that the smoking rates at Job Corps were problematic, even though their respective reasons for thinking so were different. Family Education Diabetes Series (FEDS; see Chapter 2) participants agreed that diabetes was a serious personal and community problem, although rationales behind concerns varied across group roles (e.g., patients, family members, providers, agency administrators). The young men in the Relationships Project described in Chapter 8 readily agreed on the importance of key relationships in their school as influences on their academic success. Getting this buy-in may sound like an obvious strategy, but too often professionals see a problem that a community is not focused on enough to sustain momentum. Establishing shared investment means that "we are in this together" for the long haul. This sets the stage for everyone involved to contribute their respective and unique energy and resources to the project. It's important that no one person is driving a project forward and pulling others along to make it work. If they do, then when that person tires or the grant ends, so does the project.

Secure Institutional Buy-In

Most community projects are housed within some type of institution. Whether a local school, clinic, hospital, church, or social service agency, these institutions' public visibility serves as a credibility card for the groups' efforts. They also tend to offer the brick-and-mortar locations for initial and ongoing meetings (from small ones with action-and-planning forums to large public launches) and startup resources. And because citizen health care projects are almost invariably slow in their formation and planning phases, administrators must buy into, be patient with, and otherwise support something for a long time that—from the outside in—may seem like a considerable risk of time and resources.

An institutional champion, then, with influence to make space available, provide for small startup expenses, and buffer against naysayers within the setting is essential. Some of these champions, in our experience, have been active members of the citizen health care projects themselves (e.g., Partners in Diabetes, FEDS, the Relationships Project, the Como Clinic Health Club). Others have believed in the work but were less directly involved (e.g., SANTA, the Police and Black Men Project). But they were always key to projects' survival. We have found, too, that without an institutional champion, even after an initiative has matured (as with the Como Clinic Health Club), the likelihood of that project continuing long-term is in peril.

Be Careful About External Funding, Especially at the Outset

A common expectation in academia and some community organizations is that no project should commence until the originators secure external funding. These monies directly compensate professionals for their time and cover purchases for necessary equipment, space, and other resources while simultaneously supporting the institution through indirect monies. Professionals' and agency leaders' competence and contributions are generally evaluated by the number of grant dollars secured or professional papers published (more, even, than the real-world outcomes of the projects).

A downside of these traditionally planned and funded projects is that there is often limited opportunity for cocreation by members of communities. The limited time between the grant announcement and the grant application often requires that professionals make the key decisions about projects' design and evaluation. Once the project is funded, its preestablished timelines and deliverables mean that the professionals drive the project in consultation with community members but not in deep partnership with them. This process makes it highly unlikely that the project will continue after the grant ends. On the other hand, sometimes funders will accept unusual conditions such as a great deal of flexibility in the grant development timeline and in the execution of the project that do not undermine deep community partnerships. As professionals and community members begin conversations about shared pressure points, then, they do so without time pressures to "create something" prematurely and expectations that the project itself will necessarily unfold in the manner outlined in the proposal.

With this cautionary backdrop in mind, we are aware that universities and community agencies need to financially survive. Many of our projects have gotten started as part of professionals' pro bono community outreach or service efforts that are allowed and encouraged by our university. We learned that while generating revenue through seeing clients or securing external grants to support other work (as part of our day job), we could begin to engage in conversations with community members about shared pressure points that everyone can address. If everyone contributes from the first idea onward, then the project idea is less likely to dissolve if external funding is not available at the moment.

Aim for Transformed Civic Identities

We have stressed elsewhere in this book (see the Introduction and Chapter 1) that becoming a citizen therapist involves adding a new identity. Just as professionals have been socialized as experts to identify and solve problems, community members (laypersons) are socialized to be passive recipients of professionals' expertise and to follow professional leaders in any groups that they may join. The citizen health care process invites community members, including clients or patients, to buy into the notion that they are public problem solvers and not just recipients of services. This is an identify shift, an expansion of how they see themselves in the world. They become civic actors, citizen parents, citizen teens, and patient leaders. When this civic identity transformation occurs, these community members do not easily let a project fail.

An example: In the Partners in Diabetes project (described in the introduction to this book), an early effort to host a launch event was almost derailed when we ran out of chairs in the clinic's waiting room during its setup process the night before the event. Instead of presuming that the professionals would somehow find or rent chairs, the community participants volunteered to bring folding chairs from their own basements or garages. Later in the project, when clinic resources got overwhelmed with sending out flyers to advertise a diabetes-related health fair, community participants worked with clinic staff to fill and stamp envelopes for a mass mailing. Why? Because they had internalized the project goals and taken on the identity as citizen patients.

The FEDS (see Chapter 2) has functioned over the past 20-plus years in a similar manner, with lean times and times of plenty in terms of external resources. When the project has had funding, food served during community forums is arguably more varied and plentiful. But when it has not had funding, the forums continued with food supplied by participants, potluck style. With funding, the FEDS has used sophisticated pre–post assays of participants' metabolic functioning; without funding, participants have continued to vigilantly track basic health data related to weight and body mass index (these do not cost anything to measure). Again, the participants saw it as their project and saw themselves as community change agents.

Identify Leaders and Then More Leaders

Part of the job of any professional or community member in a citizen health care project is to think about who will replace them when they are gone. Sometimes we can predict the future (e.g., a professional's changing work situation or impending retirement, a young person's graduation), and other times we cannot predict it (e.g., health emergencies, job loss), but we all know that change and transitions are a constant. At the heart of a sustainable project, then, is a concerted effort to seek out, find, nurture, and prepare people who have leadership potential and abilities.

We have done this in a variety of ways over the years. In the FEDS initiative, Elders and other participants have identified new, well-respected, visible, and trusted community members. We have invited them to take part in the FEDS, learn about it, and consider assuming leadership roles if they are inclined to. Many have. In the SANTA initiative (see Chapter 3), students in the leadership group worked to nominate younger students with strong investments in health paired with engaging and collaborative dispositions to take their place when they (the older students) graduated. The Como Clinic Health Club (see Chapter 4), during its 12 years of operation, had three "generations" of citizen patient leaders, although two individuals were involved since the founding.

Across these projects, there is usually some kind of overlap in old and new leaders' involvement. This serves to effectively pass the baton so that group leadership is seamless, while providing time to orient new leaders through meetings and project events. When everyone involved believes in the work and is invited into leadership, they want the project to last longer than their own time in it; they want it to reach more people than they will personally meet and know.

Be Patient With Program Development

Citizen health care projects, by their nature, take time to develop—time to hear all voices and to gather information about the pressure points and existing resources in the community and local institutions. They take time to envision and create interventions that involve both professionals' and community members' wisdom and contributions. They take time to go back to the drawing board when things do not work out or when revisions and refinements are necessary after evaluations show the need for change.

In other words, these projects can be slow and methodical during their gestation periods and initial rollouts. This fact must be shared and normalized with everyone involved. To both professional and community participants, we say something like, "Navigate the journey, do it together, and enjoy it. Let it unfold at its own pace. Come on board if you feel you can be patient with a process that is slow to develop and then powerful in execution." After learning to be this clear with professionals and community members who express initial interest in a project, we moved past early experiences, such as what happened in Putting Family First (see Chapter 5) in its startup phase when some leadership group members complained at every meeting about wanting quick action. More than a decade later at the launch of the Police and Black Men Project (see Chapter 9), Bill explicitly told the police officers and community members being recruited that they should expect a year of conversation and trust building before the group would take action.

Be Careful (Always!) About the Pull of the Traditional Provider–Consumer Model

We have found over the years that when citizen health care projects encounter times of duress (e.g., the space for a planned community event is suddenly not available, an original deadline for getting mailings sent out to community members is coming up too fast), professionals can feel pulled to fix, rescue, or otherwise resolve the problem without involving other community members. It's what is expected of professionals in our day jobs. However, professionals' efforts to save the day in citizen health care projects can backfire and sabotage the viability and sustainability of the work. Not involving community collaborators in problem solving undermines the democratic process and the mutual trust essential in this work. It would be better to delay a community event until a new location was collaboratively found—or to get mailings out later than originally planned—than to unilaterally fix something and then tell community partners how you did this. It's okay to slow down and to remember that everyone is in this work together and that leadership is a shared role in a flattened hierarchy.

Create Ways to Fold New Learnings Back Into the Community

All learnings, whether they come from the lived experience and wisdom of community members or the graduate training of professionals, can become the shared "property" of a citizen initiative. This information can represent a resource for all participants in a group (present and future). Internet chat rooms, web pages, social media platforms, hardcopy informational pamphlets, and booklets are all examples of ways to do this. It is important, too, to allow community participants to create and maintain these; professionals can sabotage the group if they jump in to do it for them, equipped with their technical knowledge or baseline workplace resources.

Forge a Sense of Larger Purpose

At the same time that a citizen group works pragmatically to create local interventions and engage local community members, it is important to remember the larger BHAG (big, hairy, audacious goal) that drives it. This work is about activated citizens changing the world, starting with their own community. The FEDS, for example, is not just about improving the health of the participants who take part in it. The FEDS aspires to eliminate health disparities that plague Indigenous people. The narrative statement of the Police and Black Men Project was aimed at the national challenge of relations between the police and the Black community. A sense of serving a larger purpose is crucial to keeping a project alive for many years. There are moments in meetings when it works for the citizen therapist/process leader to be deliberately inspirational, as when Bill once said, "We are trying to change health care in America!" and a group member responded, "That's too modest. We are trying to change the world!"

Obsess About Effective Group Process

A downside of democratic process is the tendency to have unfocused and undisciplined meetings. This leads community members and professionals alike to become frustrated, skip meetings, and drop out. Highly effective meeting planning and facilitation are essential for keeping people engaged in a project over many years. In our experience, it's common for group members to say that these are the best meetings they have ever participated in. We've learned to facilitate in a way to get everyone's voice into the discussion and also get things done. Once the group decides on something (like the wording of the problem being addressed or a specific action step to be taken), it's written down and becomes a record that the group reads through at subsequent meetings.

In group process, seemingly small things mean a lot for the endurance of a group. For example, we end meetings on time. This allows community members to tell their loved ones when they expect to be home—and to follow through. (Parents of young children have repeatedly praised ending meetings on time!) In addition, citizen health care meetings have written agendas that have desired outcomes for the meeting and a realistic plan for meeting those outcomes. We evolved a check-in question that gets everyone into the meeting process: "What's on your mind about our work together?" Our check-out question invites an evaluation of the meeting process and outcomes: "How do you feel about our work in this meeting?" For a decade, Bill kept notes on how group members answered this check-out question. The most common word used by community members across projects was "excited." That's because the work was important to them, and the process worked.

CONCLUSION

Although there is nothing wrong with brief projects that make a difference in a community, we have generally favored projects that last for years because the issues or pressure points being tackled have long histories and require sustained efforts. This approach allows for community ownership of the project and for the development of expanded identities among the participants. It allows for identifying and correcting mistakes and for cycles of evaluation that lead to improved interventions. In Chapter 12 we turn to this topic of evaluation.

12

FUNDING AND EVALUATION IN CITIZEN HEALTH CARE

In Chapter 11, we described a number of strategies for sustaining collaborative projects over the long haul. In this chapter, we describe ways that funding can be secured to support such projects. We then discuss ways to evaluate projects that are consistent with citizen health care principles.

STRATEGIES, RESPONSIBILITIES, AND OPTICS OF GRANT WRITING

For all of our warnings about securing external funding too early, we are not naïve about the value of financial support for projects. Especially after a project is off the ground, external funding can represent an important driver of continued backing by the agency that houses the project, ongoing functioning of the project, various forms of evaluation, and administrative benchmarks of job performance for citizen professionals involved in the project. More specifically, while host agencies oftentimes will accommodate professionals' time and donate space during a project's early phases, external funding to pay for

https://doi.org/10.1037/0000378-013
Becoming a Citizen Therapist: Integrating Community Problem-Solving Into Your Work as a Healer, by W. J. Doherty and T. J. Mendenhall

that time and space is helpful later as a way to sustain that support. As projects advance, external funding is often key in paying for food and refreshments and intervention supplies (e.g., information pamphlets, handouts and copying, office materials, medical tests, provisions). Evaluating interventions usually costs money, and securing external funding can be a marker of good work performance for the citizen professional.

Building on this last point, we recommend that professionals in community agencies and professionals in academic institutions coordinate their grant-writing efforts in purposeful ways. Resource grants (to cover things such as space and intervention supplies) are best led by community agency personnel because they are generally better informed about local and regional opportunities. They are also better ambassadors for the project to local community funders. Research grants (to support project evaluations, project improvements, and dissemination of findings) are best led by academic personnel because they are generally better informed about foundation, state, and federal opportunities. They are also better positioned to present themselves as credentialed investigators, and their university will have an infrastructure, including an institutional review board and secure data storage, to support research and evaluation.

No matter who is formally designated as the lead, we have found that the optics of partnering across community and academic sectors as coinvestigators or coprincipal investigators make for ideal competitiveness for funding. Community agencies applying for funds are more competitive if a university entity is working with them to advance and evaluate the work that they are doing. In turn, academicians are more competitive when it is clear that leaders of that community are working closely with them to house, organize, and otherwise sustain the project. Everybody wins.

EVALUATION PROCESSES IN CITIZEN HEALTH CARE

In traditional community projects, evaluation is largely determined by professionals who are seen as experts in connecting the goals of the project to measures of outcomes. Professionals generally take the lead in data analysis, interpretation, and dissemination (publications, presentations, media reports, etc.) without meaningful community involvement (Berge et al., 2009; D'Alonzo, 2010; Krishnan et al., 2020). In citizen health care projects, professionals and lay community members work collaboratively over time to plan and carry out evaluation efforts. This is important to understand because evaluation does not always mean straightforward pre–posttests of an established project's outcome. Though we certainly do this type of evaluation in our projects, it is not the only evaluation we do. Following are other important forms of evaluation.

Formative Evaluation

Formative evaluation involves assessing how a new program can be appropriate or feasible within a community (Nieveen & Folmer, 2013; Powell, 2006; Salabarría-Peña et al., 2007). This is important to do early on because it can inform programming logistics and modifications before a new initiative publicly launches and thereby maximizes the likelihood that professional–community collaborations will be successful. In Putting Family First and Play It Forward! (see Chapter 5), the leadership group did extensive interviewing in the community to assess whether the formulation of the problem and the initial plans would be desired and feasible.

Process (Implementation) Evaluation

Process evaluations represent efforts to determine if a project is moving forward in the way intended (Erkens, 2019; Moore et al., 2015). This helps ensure consistency between a project design and its delivery (e.g., its accessibility to community members), and it can identify reasons to shift gears. The Como Clinic Health Club (see Chapter 4) initially developed and piloted a format for a collaborative goal-setting session between patients and their primary care clinicians, but process evaluation of its feasibility uncovered insurance and scheduling problems. The group decided to shift to activities that did not involve these logistical challenges.

Outcome (Effectiveness) and Impact Evaluations

Outcome evaluations are designed to assess whether a program is effective in achieving the objectives that its designers set out to accomplish (Friedman et al., 2021; Grembowski, 2015). These efforts can begin as soon as an initiative is formally launched by tracking measurements relevant to participants' reasons for taking part in the program. The Family Education Diabetes Series (FEDS; see Chapter 2) has many examples of outcome evaluation, both medical and psychosocial.

Impact evaluations assess program outcomes in a more definitive and final way, such as whether the overall rate of a problem has declined in a specific community (Bryant-Lukosius et al., 2016; Clarke et al., 2019). Although we have not done impact evaluations as of 2023, one is in the planning stages for Braver Angels (see Chapter 7) as that project begins to address polarization at the community level and evaluate it via polling of community members before a variety of interventions and several years later to see if there has been a global change in polarized attitudes relative to a control community that does not receive the interventions.

COMMUNITY-BASED PARTICIPATORY RESEARCH

In our citizen health care initiatives, we usually follow principles of outcome evaluation that are consistent with community-based participatory research. This approach is also called action research, participatory research, participatory action research, and other names that vary by professional discipline (e.g., Brush et al., 2020; Israel et al., 2005; McIntyre, 2008; Stringer & Aragon, 2021). The most important of these principles are addressed in this section.

Collaboratively Define Project Outcomes

Engage with community members at the outset regarding what the desired outcomes of an initiative are. These conversations will help to guide the larger focus and pragmatic steps of the intervention in a manner ensuring that all voices are honored and will serve to get members thinking together about how to assess whether and in what ways that intervention is successful. Sometimes unanimous agreement will be evident (in the Family Education Diabetes Series, weight, body mass index [BMI], and metabolic control have been consistently agreed upon). Other times professionals will be especially interested in something (e.g., assessment via food diaries) while community members are interested in something else (e.g., change in a local school's policy about whether to allow a child with diabetes to go on field trips with their peers). As the group decides together what to measure, all members become invested in the outcomes.

Collaboratively Decide on Data Collection and Management Methods

After outcomes are collectively articulated, it is not automatically the professionals' job to decide how to gather data, nor is it wholly their job to do the data gathering. Instead, the full leadership group decides these things together via questions and conversations. Here are some examples of questions from FEDS meetings:

- How should we measure weight? With a standardized beam scale? Should we use just one, or several? If we use several, how can we ensure that they are synchronized?

- Should professionals record weight data, or should community members do that? And if it is community members, should they record their own data or only others' data?

- Metabolic control is measured with blood draws, so professionals should do that—right?

- BMI can be calculated online once we know a person's weight and height, so community members can do that—right?

- What about qualitative data, like key-informant interviews? What questions should we ask? What does everyone want to know? What are some things that only some of us want to know?

- Should qualitative interviews be conducted by folks with formal training about how to do them? Can community members be trained to do these interviews, or should it only be professionals who conduct them? Who is going to transcribe all of the recordings?

Questions such as these move groups toward a constellation of methods that have everyone's input and involvement. Some data are collected by professionals only. Other data are collected by community members only. Other data, still, can be collected by anybody.

The process of data management, too, should be collaboratively determined. In our experience, the actual work is done by graduate students under senior professionals' supervision, but only after discussions with and permission from the group. And it is not uncommon for community members to serve as spot-checkers of quantitative data entry or transcribed qualitative interviews to ensure both accuracy and (more importantly) co-ownership of a group's database.

Collaboratively Analyze and Interpret Data

Professionals usually lead efforts in data analysis. They tend to be more conversant with statistical platforms such as SPSS and SAS for quantitative data and more skilled with tests to assess a program's effectiveness over time and in comparison with other programs or control groups. Professionals similarly tend to be more familiar with platforms such as NVivo or Quirkos for the analysis of qualitative data derived from key-informant interviews, talking circles, field observations, documents, and related records.

On the other hand, it is essential to include community members in interpreting what findings are drawn. For example, are nonsignificant comparisons between two groups a good thing or a bad thing? Are statistically significant differences between two time points within one group (e.g., via a single-group, repeated-measures design) or between two groups in comparison to each other (e.g., via a randomized controlled trial) really about the intervention or about something else in the shared environment that was not expected but happened anyway? Are common narratives across multiple interviews indicative of a pathology within the group or something else, even a strength not well-expressed? Are common themes related to success unique to intervention participants or are these themes happening everywhere in the local community?

In sum, involving community members in data interpretation is essential to establishing confidence in how results are understood and then disseminated across both professional and community audiences.

Collaboratively Disseminate Study Findings

Many communities—especially minority communities—have long-standing histories of being researched by professionals who leave after collecting data, often never to come back (Goodman et al., 2018; Neufeld et al., 2019; Sukarieh & Tanhock, 2013). The professionals benefit from the work (e.g., dissertations, refereed publications, guild presentations, promotion, tenure), but the communities often do not. In citizen health care initiatives, we try to disseminate findings across both professional and lay community audiences and do this in ways that showcase the collaborative nature of the work.

Peer-reviewed journal articles, for example, are the principal currency of academic professionals' success. However, few people outside of academia read—or even have access to—these publications, and direct benefits to the communities involved are hard to detect. On the other hand, community publications such as local newspapers and pamphlets, websites accessed by community members, and presentations at local powwows and health fairs directly reach the people who have been the focus of the project. The products of this work benefit the sponsoring agency of the initiative in terms of its visibility, reach, credibility, and competitiveness for future local grants. However, such publications and presentations do little to help researchers in traditional academic settings.

And so, again: Citizen health care initiatives work hard to honor both professional and community audiences as they disseminate the work. These dissemination efforts often mean academic publications and presentations along with community-based outlets. Either way, it's important that professional and community members of the leadership team coauthor and copresent, with their names strategically positioned with the audience in mind. This way, everybody involved benefits with the audiences they most care about.

Iteratively Respond to Ongoing Evaluation Data

It is common to see published literature that describes a one-time evaluation of an intervention. It is often not clear if or how the original intervention was revised in response to initial outcome data; in other words, is the current evaluation based on revisions from prior learnings in the project? In citizen health care initiatives, it is important to engage in iterative cycles of project evaluation and refinement, with or without formal funding, and even if professional journals reject sequential submissions for publication because earlier manuscripts of what they see as the same study have been published. However, ongoing data collection is a powerful way to inform how a project is doing and in what ways it should continue, revise, stop, or add intervention components to do even better.

The FEDS is our best example of this iterative process. Over more than 20 years, we have evaluated the intervention's effectiveness across biological, psychological, and social dependent variables. We have conducted multiple qualitative queries into participants' perceptions about key program influences on quantitative outcomes formally measured. In response to data collected, we have modified programming to include more attention to selected health topics (e.g., stress management, reading food labels) and less attention to other topics (e.g., diabetes' effects on vision). We have increased small-group activities (e.g., talking circles), live demonstrations (e.g., chair aerobics), and large-group games (e.g., diabetes bingo). We have eliminated previous teachings about wound care, and we have added new teachings about historical trauma, anxiety, and depression.

At the time of this writing, we estimate that the FEDS has undergone several dozen tests and analyses of outcome data. However, a formal search reveals just five refereed journal articles about the program (Berge et al., 2009; Doherty et al., 2010; Doherty & Mendenhall, 2006; Mendenhall et al., 2010; Seal et al., 2016), alongside three more descriptive book chapters (Mendenhall et al., 2013, 2018; Mendenhall, Berge, & Doherty, 2014), three trade articles (Doherty et al., 2014; Mendenhall, 2021; Mendenhall, Doherty, et al., 2008), and 17 professional presentations. Community publications and publications, of course, are not searchable in the same manner. But this is okay! The point is that our evaluations are ongoing even if they do not get formally shared with the rest of the world. Because with each iteration, the FEDS has improved, along with its likelihood for survival through buy-in by professional and community stakeholders alike and through buy-in by new and veteran members alike.

CONCLUSION

Evaluation will differ for every citizen therapist project. Some evaluations will be intensive and systematic and others more informal. But asking the questions about how we are doing our work and what difference we are making is essential to mindful community engagement projects. Notice that the key word here is *we*: How do we do project evaluation together, knowing that the needs and interests of professionals and other community members align in some ways and differ in other ways? When common and differing interests are explicit and on the table, evaluation becomes a rewarding part of work.

13 GETTING STARTED AS A CITIZEN THERAPIST

In prior chapters we described a wide range of citizen therapist projects. Now it's time to discuss how you can initiate your own project if the work appeals to you. This chapter offers strategies for choosing an issue to focus on, for engaging a community, and for recruiting a partnership organization or institution. We also share lessons learned from citizen health care projects that failed to get traction because of mistakes in the startup phase.

For most therapists learning to do citizen therapist projects, the work will involve a volunteer commitment of time, especially in early stages, although some projects might be funded. In either case, being a citizen therapist (as we envision it) is not a full-time job that takes you away from your clinical work or day job. Rather, it involves the expansion of your professional horizon to make a difference at the community level and to do so in a disciplined way.

https://doi.org/10.1037/0000378-014
Becoming a Citizen Therapist: Integrating Community Problem-Solving Into Your Work as a Healer, by W. J. Doherty and T. J. Mendenhall

THE ISSUE MUST FEEL PERSONALLY AND PROFESSIONALLY REWARDING TO WORK ON

Creating a citizen therapist project should not feel like another obligation or something that pulls you away from what you most enjoy doing. It's akin to choosing a dissertation topic: You must be interested enough in the area to sustain a couple of years of effort. So, ask what's your personal and professional energy for an issue and how working on it dovetails with your self-interest. The question of self-interest is seldom asked of graduate students and professionals, and it can seem a bit, well, nonprofessional and self-serving. After all, professionals are supposed to be objective and set aside self-interest as they help people or pursue research knowledge. In every graduate class where students present their research interests, Bill has them answer these questions: What is your personal interest in pursuing this research topic? And how does your choice of this topic relate to your background, different identities, and goals for your career? Students often struggle with the questions because they've never been asked them, but they report benefiting from tackling them because doing so is clarifying.

If you want to entertain the idea of citizen therapist work, it's good to begin with your main clinical interests, particularly ones that engage you personally. As therapists, we know our choice of clinical interests is not random. We are attracted to psychological and relational issues because they appeal to us in some way. Sometimes we've struggled with the issue ourselves or have seen it affect our family. In one class, a student was interested in how families deal with suicide, and another student focused on culturally sensitive therapy for African immigrants. Both students had no trouble articulating their personal reasons for dedicating themselves to studying these issues. Another student, though, initially struggled with the question. She wanted to study socioemotional learning in middle schools. At first her response to the self-interest question stayed at the level of research gaps—why a specific focus on middle schools would enhance that research and eventually help kids. Bill kept asking why that was important to her, and eventually the student talked movingly about how inadequate she had felt as a teacher when she could not help kids with their emotional and social lives. That experience gave her passion for the work.

For us (Bill and Tai), our self-interest came out of dissatisfaction with the impact of our clinical work alone on public problems that keep getting worse. Bill was also tired of trying to improve health care by changing how physicians engaged with patients and families. Economic forces in health care proved to be more powerful influences on physician behavior than anything he taught. He also worried that just training more therapists would not make the larger world better. As described in the introduction (this book), Bill was on fire to try something different after he learned about citizen professionalism. In that sense, the specific issue was not as important as the opportunity to break out of the constraints of traditional professionalism and engage in democratic renewal with communities—and to offer leadership in the field.

For his part, Tai was feeling increasingly frustrated with how all the success stories he was learning about in his classes (if the therapist—generally isolated in a private practice—just chose the right theory, advanced the right approach, or said the right things) continually did not manifest in the work he was doing in a busy primary care clinic. And as he collaborated with providers representing a myriad of other disciplines, he remained dissatisfied by the paucity of patients' and families' voice and participation in the care and adaptation to chronic conditions that they were navigating. He also felt constrained by his inability to connect patients with other patients; they had much to offer each other but instead were made to not embrace this desire to help secondary to Health Insurance Portability and Accountability Act (HIPAA) rules. In that sense and like Bill's story, the specific issue (e.g., diabetes, chronic pain) was not as important as the opportunity to engage in democratic action in which communities and providers work together.

PRIORITIZE ISSUES WHERE PEOPLE NEED WAYS TO CONNECT

Citizen therapist work is all about facilitating mutual teaching and learning among people dealing with life challenges. Therefore, the best issues for projects are likely to be ones where there are few structures in place for people to form and sustain these peer connections. An example of a good connection structure already in place is Alcoholics Anonymous. Likewise, individuals and families facing some chronic illnesses in children have similar support mechanisms (examples are muscular dystrophy and hemophilia). The same is true in some areas of the disability community, where online groups have become particularly important. But for many other health and social challenges, there are limited opportunities for people to connect, learn from each other, and try to make a difference in their community. We started with diabetes in the American Indian community partly for that reason: It was (is) a high-impact health problem with few community supports and connections in place.

In sum, ask yourself about the current opportunities for people dealing with your main clinical interest to connect with one another and consider the quality of these opportunities (e.g., some online communities are more helpful than others).

FAVOR PRESSURE POINT ISSUES FOR AN IDENTIFIABLE COMMUNITY

The issue you engage with cannot be something that professionals care about a lot more than community members do. (An example is spanking or corporal punishment, which appears to concern professionals more than it does many communities.) We repeat: It must be something that troubles a community— or what we call a pressure point. Diabetes in the American Indian community and overscheduled kids in a suburban mostly White community were pressure points, as was policing for an urban Black community.

The issue must also be a pressure point for professionals: something they worry about and know they can't handle without deep cooperation with individuals and communities. Heart transplants are not a professional pressure point for surgeons and cardiologists (other than getting enough funding), whereas diabetes and tobacco use are areas of frustration for many physicians, just as public safety and community support for policing are major pressure points for public safety professionals.

Furthermore, the community can't be "the world." It has to be a group who can identify as a "we," often a community of concern about a health or social issue. It could also involve a geographic community (like American Indians in Ramsey County, Minnesota, or police and Black men in Minneapolis). It could be a virtual community with no geographic boundaries. None of our own projects have been done with online communities, but we see that as a new frontier for citizen therapist work.

START WITH A COMMUNITY WHERE YOU HAVE CONNECTIONS

Don't go searching for a community in need where you know almost no one and have built no trust. Look first at communities that you are part of and have credibility in. This can be the community where you work, study, or live or an online community that you are part of. For Bill's early project with Putting Family First, he had credibility from having given presentations in Wayzata and from writing a book that some residents had read.

If you do not already have connections, develop a relationship with a community leader who can sponsor you. That's where you will find out what the pressure points are and whether there is overlap between your interests and that of the community. The process of developing a sponsoring relationship can take many months or even years and often involves showing up at community events and following up with people your sponsor introduces you to. For Tai, this happened in the American Indian community when two

Elders who knew him from his work in Partners in Diabetes vouched for him. For Bill, doctoral student Corey Yeager sponsored his introduction to the Office of Black Male Student Achievement, where Corey worked.

IF YOU ARE CONSIDERING A LONG-TERM PROJECT, RECRUIT A COMMUNITY ORGANIZATION

Over a series of 20 or so projects, we have learned that ones that take place outside of a sponsoring organization tend to have a life expectancy of 2 to 3 years, whereas ones that are housed and sponsored by a community organization or institution tend to last longer. As discussed in Chapter 11 (this book), a sponsoring organization can provide basic logistical support (e.g., meeting space, copy machine) and some staff coordination time (usually written into a staff member's job description). And if the organization has a steady stream of clients or patients, it also provides a pool from which new citizen leaders can emerge for the project as the initial leaders move on. Projects outside of a sponsoring organization usually finish up when the initial leaders feel they have accomplished something meaningful.

The following are strategies for recruiting a community organization (such as a medical clinic, a social service agency, or a school) to a citizen therapist project:

- Connect your idea to the mission of the organization. For example, the Como Clinic was part of HealthPartners, whose mission statement refers to promoting the health of the community.

- Connect your idea to a pressure point for the organization, something they wish they were doing better with. Diabetes was a big concern for the Interfaith Action of Greater Saint Paul's Department of Indian Work, as was smoking for the Hubert H. Humphrey Job Corps. The Minneapolis Police Department was eager to improve community ties.

- Engage senior leadership to enhance the likelihood of longevity as staff members turn over. In one project, we dealt only with midlevel professional staff, and when they departed the project ended. In subsequent projects, we learned to get buy-in at the highest staff level, particularly the CEO.

- Engage with frontline staff who would like to learn how to partner deeply with community members. It is crucial that the professional staff participants see the project as enhancing their own careers and skills.

- Make sure that everyone understands the slow, developmental nature of the project so that you are not blindsided by a supervisor who has different expectations. A colleague working on a project had a new supervisor who kept questioning her about why the project was developing so slowly. The project never took off. We should have met with the staff member and her new supervisor to orient her to the nature of this work.

DEVELOP A FOCUS FOR THE PROJECT BEFORE RECRUITING CITIZEN LEADERS

We have learned that a project leadership group can get bogged down in choosing a focus and then lose energy for the action stage. This happened with a project in which a colleague learning the citizen health care model engaged with a group of parents who were concerned about the over-sexualization of young girls in our society. Group members differed from the beginning about whether to focus on traditional gender expectations (pink and Barbie dolls) or on the more blatant sexualization of girls' clothing and other commercial appeals to grow up fast. After many months of discussion with no clarity about a focus or preliminary action plans, the group finally dissolved. In retrospect, because the citizen therapist leader was mainly interested in the commercial sexualization aspect, it would have been better to recruit parents who were interested in focusing there.

An example where we did better was a project with the Liberian immigrant community in the northern suburbs of Minneapolis. The focus that was mutually agreed upon at the outset was on the lingering effects of war and trauma, not broader issues of immigrant stress or ongoing legal struggles over refugee status. Similarly, with the Como Clinic Health Club, the group agreed from the beginning on the boundary that Bill proposed as consistent with the citizen health care model: We would not be recommending any changes in health care delivery in the clinics. Our focus would be on how we could create a health-promoting community of patients, not on how providers do their job. The group readily accepted the boundary, which kept the project from turning into a traditional advisory group, a path that generally leads to professional leaders explaining to less informed patients why changes they suggest are not feasible.

In sum, it should be clear from the first recruitment efforts what issue you will be working on. People self-select into projects based on their interests and passions. Then the process of cocreation begins.

BE INTENTIONAL ABOUT HOW MUCH TIME YOU SPEND ON THE PROJECT

It is tempting to overfunction as a citizen therapist when you are excited about a project. This can lead you to do work that other citizens should be doing. A classic motto of community organizing is to "never say what someone else can say, and never do what someone else can do." As citizen therapists, Tai and Bill generally work about 8 hours per month on a project—a couple of hours per week. The time commitment is more longitudinal (over years) rather than intensive week by week.

We stress these time limitations for citizen therapist volunteers when their main livelihood is clinical work. If you are a staff member in clinic, you should negotiate the specific amount of time that you can spend on a project and how it will fit with your other professional responsibilities. As university faculty members, we have done our citizen therapist work as part of our (required) community outreach, with the time commitment being extensive over years (rather than, again, intensively week by week), although there can be specific periods of lots of time on project activities. We have put in additional time writing grants and articles, all within our faculty roles.

If you are a graduate student, the time commitment is particularly important to balance with the regular requirements of your program. If you are doing a project for course credit, make sure that your faculty member understands that the learning objectives are adapted to the evolutionary nature of citizen health care projects. Finally, because project timelines are outside of your control and because the project could take a different direction than anticipated, we urge caution about doing a citizen health care project for a master's thesis or doctoral dissertation. Evaluating an ongoing project, though, might work well for a thesis or dissertation.

LESSONS FROM OUR STARTUP MISTAKES

Earlier we referred to a project that never took off because its focus at the outset was uncertain, and the group's energy for action waned as it took such a long time to agree on that focus. Some members were deflated about the prospect of not having their preference reflected in the group's mission. If the Family Education Diabetes Series had begun without clarity that its focus was on diabetes, it might have had a similar fate, given the myriad of health problems recognized as threatening in the American Indian community.

As mentioned, there is a lot of room for preliminary work to determine which community pressure point to work on in a project. This determination can come from one-to-one conversations with community members and from consulting with organizational leaders who might sponsor a project. Again: no pressure point, no project. But we have learned the hard way that once recruitment begins for citizen leaders, there should be clarity about which problem or issue they are being invited to tackle together.

Another mistake we've made is to proceed with too few community members in the leadership group. An example was a project where we were training "citizen librarians" in how to initiate a citizen professional project based in a county library that attracted a large immigrant population, particularly parents and young children, as patrons. As with most libraries, there was no vehicle to engage parents in the library's mission to promote literacy and reading skills. Patrons come just as consumers of library services. After embracing the idea of a citizen professional approach, the librarians did one-to-one interviews with parents who regularly brought their children to the library. From those interviews they pulled together a group of four motivated immigrant parents whose children regularly used the library. Perhaps because getting this project off the ground took so many months, and the sponsoring county administrators were impatient to see results, we failed to urge the citizen librarians to spend enough time to triple the number of parents in the initial leadership group. (The ideal citizen leadership group size is 12–15 citizens, small enough for deliberation but large enough to accommodate inevitable attrition in the early stages.) Instead, a small group of four parents and two librarians began to plan their first outreach project. When two of the parents pulled out because of family problems (a sick child, a new job), the group became too small to launch the project. Two lessons here: Wait until you have an adequate number of citizen leaders, and if you can't attract at least 12, maybe the project idea is not engaging the community in a powerful enough way. Better to go back to the drawing board than to start with too few citizen leaders.

Another example targeted depression among immigrant and refugee men in a local Hmong community. Providers at a primary care clinic were wholly on board with this pressure point, insofar as they saw depression as a clinical presentation that was both widespread and generally unresponsive to medication or talk therapies. Initial conversations (through interpreters) suggested that several patients shared in this investment to do something, but early meetings to discuss and launch a citizen therapist project were repeatedly derailed by a mismatch between professionals' and community members' narratives. Whereas professionals focused on creating an outward-facing project to allay depression in the Hmong community, patients approached the meetings more like conventional group therapy. Over the course of several conversations within the larger group (and between smaller groups of professional leaders and interpreters), it became clear that the men would not feel comfortable engaging in a public manner around a highly sensitive issue such as depression. In retrospect, this misstep could have been avoided if the professionals had more thoroughly understood cultural stigmas attached to depression and if they had explored the citizen health care idea more thoroughly with community members (and likely then decided to not proceed) before prematurely charging forward.

CONCLUDING THOUGHTS

This chapter has covered startup strategies. These will be effective only in light of what we address in the next chapter: the self-identity of the citizen therapist. Our work as citizen therapists is not just to be strategically competent but to inspire confidence that the democratic, cocreative process of conversation, mutual influence, and consultation with other citizens will pay off for everyone involved. This is a countercultural way of working that we've seen people end up loving—but it can feel strange at first. A main part of leadership for the citizen therapist is to show the way for a new kind of working relationship with communities and their citizens.

14 THE CITIZEN THERAPIST AS A PERSON AND AS A PROFESSIONAL

In Chapter 13, we wrote about professional dissatisfactions that led us to citizen therapist work. We were each frustrated with the scope and reach of our work as clinicians and academics. (Recall the provocatively titled book *We've Had a Hundred Years of Psychotherapy and the World's Getting Worse* [Hillman & Ventura, 1993]). You may not feel similarly frustrated or dissatisfied, but perhaps you have an itch to get involved in something beyond your day job that makes a difference in your community or the larger world. In this chapter, we discuss the implications of citizen therapist work for the therapist as a person and professional.

HOW CITIZEN THERAPIST WORK HAS CHANGED US

We all know that doing therapy changes the therapist over time. How could this not occur over years of walking with people in their pain and hopes? Few other types of work connect people in such vulnerable and intimate ways. In almost no other profession is the self of the professional so important. In the

https://doi.org/10.1037/0000378-015
Becoming a Citizen Therapist: Integrating Community Problem-Solving Into Your Work as a Healer, by W. J. Doherty and T. J. Mendenhall

same way, becoming a citizen therapist transforms us in ways that cannot always be anticipated in advance. On the basis of our own experiences over the past 2 decades, however, we offer some ways you that may find yourself affected if you engage in citizen therapist work.

Feeling Part of Something Larger

Whereas psychotherapy is inherently private, citizen therapist work is public and social. The sense of a larger "we" from being part of a community of strivers for change is an expansive complement to clinical work (which we also value greatly). There is also a sense of connection to broader societal needs— what is happening upstream from the problems we treat in our offices—that has enlarged our purview as therapists.

This perspective applies even to areas in which we are not directly doing community work. For example, Bill has a passion for couples therapy, particularly couples on the brink of divorce or breaking up. Becoming a citizen therapist has moved him to pay more attention to the larger ecology of couples' relationships, including how poorly we prepare people to meet the historically high expectations of marriage and how the disappearance of well-paying working-class jobs has undermined marriage in so many communities. Tai has a passion for integrated health care, particularly as it relates to interdisciplinary collaboration in the support and empowerment of patients (individuals, couples, families) who are managing chronic health conditions. Becoming a citizen therapist has moved him to pay more attention to the lived experience and wisdom that patients and their loved ones possess and to include them as collaborators (drivers, even) in care. Interdisciplinary care, then, means more than a group of providers trained in different specialties working together. It means situating what we do within larger communities of expertise and thereby including the contributions of professionals with formal credentials and laypersons with in-the-trenches qualifications.

In other words, being a citizen therapist means seeing the public dimensions of all the problems that we treat in our offices and clinics. This has also affected our teaching of therapy graduate students: For every clinical topic (depression, substance abuse, couple distress, etc.), we like to begin the class discussion with a sociocultural and historical perspective: for example, how depression rates are increasing in developed countries despite the availability of more effective treatments, how social ambivalence about alcohol (disease? moral problem? social problem?) has shown itself from the 19th century temperance movement up to today's treatment modalities, and how changes in cultural norms and laws have influenced marriage and intimate relationships. Class discussions do not begin with the *Diagnostic and Statistical Manual of Mental Disorders* but instead with a larger picture. Teaching and clinical work become more expansive when you take on the identity of a citizen therapist.

A Sense of Integration Between Professional and Civic Contributions

As Boyte (2004) and Dzur (2008) have pointed out, traditional professionalism has created a division between services that we provide for individuals and how we can contribute to community or civic well-being. Health care becomes the task of professionals who, in the rest of their lives, try to be helpful as private citizens. In other words, work roles and our civic roles are non-overlapping. As professional therapists, we may volunteer at a soup kitchen, contribute money to a charitable cause, or support a candidate for office, but none of these are within our identity as a therapist. Helping the world outside of our offices is separate and distinct from our passions and expertise as therapists. This is not just an issue for our profession; it's part of a large bifurcation of work and public life, and a critique of this split gave rise to the literature on citizen professionalism.

We are reminded of the story about a bricklayer in the Middle Ages. When someone walking by asked him what he was doing as he prepared his bricks for the day, he replied, "I'm building a cathedral." (He could have just said, "I'm preparing to lay bricks today.") The cathedral would not be completed in his lifetime, but that didn't matter. As citizen therapists, we're in a public cathedral building trade, along with many other workers contributing in their own way.

Becoming a Different Kind of Expert

Both of us have had the experience of academic colleagues, after hearing us present on citizen professionalism, retort that they did not earn a PhD to pretend that they don't have expertise. This, of course, misses the mark for how we see the expertise of citizen professionals and citizen therapists. The issue is how we use our traditional expertise and how we expand our skills into new areas. For expertise in, say, depression, trauma, or coping with a medical illness, therapists bring important knowledge from research and clinical experience. The citizen therapist learns how to share this expertise in community settings via an "on tap" approach rather than an "on top" one. Among other things, this means adding one's knowledge to the mix after other citizens have contributed theirs. A citizen therapist does not hold back from sharing knowledge but is careful to not reflexively go first or employ it at the expense of other forms of knowledge from lived experience.

We have learned that the most important expertise that citizen therapists bring to citizen professional work is knowledge and skills in interpersonal behavior and group process. Facilitating meetings where everyone's voice is heard and the group gets its work done—that is a major form of expertise, as is building one-to-one relationships with community leaders and regular citizens. Interpersonal skills are particularly important when you go outside of your regular professional circle, as Tai did with the American Indian community in St. Paul and Bill did with the police community in Minneapolis.

In sum, the key expertise of citizen therapists is that of catalyst for others to come together to create work of significance in a community. Other forms of professional knowledge and expertise will come into play naturally over time, on tap, as the collective work unfolds.

More Sense of Community Connection

This is such an obvious benefit for citizen professionals that it would be easy to overlook. Citizen therapist work offers a feeling of being more widely and deeply connected to your community. The relationships are unique: They are not clinical relationships that can happen only in an office, nor are they social friendships, colleague relationships, or family bonds. The best term we know for these ties is *civic friendships*, which are relationships forged in the shared work of making the community better. Civic friends see you as a professional and appreciate your contributions, but they do not put you on a pedestal. To this point, there has always been a lot of humor in the citizen therapist projects that we have been part of, and some of that humor is directed toward the citizen therapist. Tai is teased mercilessly by his Family Education Diabetes Series (FEDS) civic friends for his lack of functioning without coffee and other assorted quirks (well-deserved, as Bill sees it), and the members of the Police and Black Men Project have a name for Bill connected with a TV commercial featuring "an old White guy" correcting people's group behavior (Tai approves). Leveling the hierarchy can take many forms that create warm bonds.

A good way to understand the differences between relationships with clients versus community members is to imagine running into people in public. With clients, most therapists are careful about acknowledging them in public because of confidentiality norms, and they don't usually introduce clients to family members in those settings. In most cases, running into a current or former client in the community is awkward for therapists, even if the clients are glad to see us. With civic relationships, it's the opposite: Everyone is glad to see one another and there are introductions all around. This happened recently for Bill outside a local coffee shop where one of the Como project leaders paused her daily walk to chat with him, and for Tai when a FEDS participant saw him and his wife while shopping at the mall.

More Joy Despite Depressing Societal Problems

There is something about working alongside fellow citizens to make a community better that inspires joy and inhibits cynicism and despair about the world we live in. In addition to the relationships formed, citizen therapist work is about collective agency to build a shared world and solve problems across diverse people and groups—and that's the essence of democracy. It's about steps we can take locally without waiting for the world to change first. It's about thinking globally and acting locally, about holding a bold vision and taking practical action. In our experience, what emerges is inspiration that leads to joy, even when projects struggle to move the needle on societal problems that appear stuck or change so slowly.

An example of this for Bill is his work on depolarizing America. The problem appears to be worse since the day he helped create Braver Angels. People around him, including his therapist colleagues and friends, are expressing pessimism and even despair about anything changing. Sometimes they pull back from politics or focus just on beating the other political party in the next election, but of course even if that happens, it's temporary satisfaction because the political system at the national level is paralyzed by division, and the other side undermines while awaiting their turn to take charge. For his part, Bill feels hopeful because he works alongside many other citizens in addressing the problem of polarization, and he sees small gains to be built upon. Hope is not so much a feeling as a choice, one that is easier to make for a citizen therapist connected to a community of action where people are not waiting for elected leaders to save us. And from hope comes joy for Bill when he witnesses moments of connection across profound political differences, when people move from demonizing to humanizing each other. He's even seen it on a small scale when working with members of Congress.

As for Tai, he finds joy in his work to eliminate health disparities in the American Indian community. At the same time, he knows that prevalence rates for a myriad of physical (e.g., diabetes, cardiovascular disease) and mental health (e.g., depression, addictions) struggles are not yet narrowing between racial–ethnic groups. Across the board, Indigenous communities appear to be faring poorly. Overwhelming social conditions (also recognized as disparities) in arenas such as income, access to high-quality education, employment, and stable housing serve to maintain or exacerbate these struggles. Historical traumas, too, associated with generations of colonization and genocide are only beginning to be widely recognized.

Given these forces, sometimes participants in the FEDS program have expressed pessimism about ever "getting better" in diabetes management, much less ever seeing larger social change. Tai, too, has struggled sometimes with not feeling like the scope of the FEDS (and like-minded offshoots) will ever reach beyond the Twin Cities metropolitan area—much less in any way that could eliminate health disparities for a whole ethnic group. But then a group participant shares in celebration that their A1C metabolic marker has improved to clinically recommended levels for the first time since being diagnosed, another shares that their physician is taking them off medication because they don't need it anymore because of significant weight loss and improved numbers, or another shares that they were suicidal until they engaged with the group. And then young persons connected to the FEDS share how they are starting a Native garden in collaboration with their school, launching an online forum for teens to access personalized resources and peer-to-peer support, and advancing a health-fair component at a large powwow. Hope emerges from resisting despair as everyone in the project celebrates small-scale successes while charging forward to larger goals that we believe will arrive someday.

LEARNING TO THINK AT TWO LEVELS AT ONCE

Just as therapists work simultaneously at the content level of what clients bring and the process level of underlying dynamics, citizen therapists function at two levels at once: on specific projects related to health or social well-being and on the process of activating and sustaining collective agency and efficacy. (That's why we put so much emphasis on leadership development.) This is especially the case for issues that have become the sole territory of professional experts or otherwise lie outside of the scope of citizen engagement. The citizen therapist aims to catalyze the energies of ordinary people not as consumers of services but as coproducers of collective solutions.

This is why, too, we say this work is about democratic renewal. The beating heart of a democracy is not just fair elections but how citizens are engaged in building the commonwealth. People who feel little agency to shape their future will turn to demagogues and divisive groups to rescue them and in the process further disempower themselves. They sometimes take undemocratic collective action against other groups whom they see as threatening. Thus, every citizen therapist project is a laboratory for developing capacity for democratic living in a diverse society, with no scapegoats and no saviors. Feeling this in our bones keeps us inspired. As Tai likes to say, even after 2 decades of this work, "We're just getting warmed up!"

AFTERWORD

In recent years it's been nearly impossible for therapists to miss the connection between their clinical offices and events and movements in the larger world. Take just three: toxic political polarization, racial reckonings after George Floyd, and the COVID pandemic. The always permeable membrane between therapy and society has become more transparent than ever before. In this book, we presented a citizen therapist approach to how to address problems that transcend clinical practice and yet deeply influence clinical practice. If you are intrigued about putting these ideas into practice, we have some final questions and thoughts for you.

First, ask yourself if you are ready to move outside of your comfort zone by engaging with community members who are not your clients. Do you have a passion, perhaps grounded in your own life or clinical interests, to work upstream from the problems that you see in your office or your own life? Not as a savior, advocate, or teacher, but as a coproducer of community work that taps the knowledge, energy, and lived experience of your fellow citizens. Not with the expectation that you will benefit financially but with confidence that the rewards will far exceed the demands on your time and energy.

https://doi.org/10.1037/0000378-016
Becoming a Citizen Therapist: Integrating Community Problem-Solving Into Your Work as a Healer, by W. J. Doherty and T. J. Mendenhall

Your fellow community members are likely to embrace your citizen therapist efforts if they tap pressure points in their lives and if you use your skills in relationship building. The challenge, in our experience, is not community interest; it's having citizen therapists and other professionals ready to provide catalytic leadership using a collaborative and disciplined approach. Come to think of it, that's what we learn to do as clinicians: use collaborative and disciplined approaches to treating clients. Our communities require nothing less of us.

That's why we are offering follow-up to this book. You can keep up with the academic and professional literature that we and others produce on citizen therapist work by accessing the website of our Citizen Professional Center at the University of Minnesota (https://innovation.umn.edu/citizen-professional-center). If you are interested in more information about how to do citizen therapist work, visit the Doherty Family Foundation for Social and Civic Well-Being (https://www.dohertyfoundation.org).

Ultimately, we want to grow a community of citizen therapists who learn together, support each other in the face of roadblocks, and expand the horizons of the field of psychotherapy. In a time of growing public division and distrust for professionals, the way forward is not to just bemoan, criticize, or stay in our traditional lane but to engage, engage, and engage.

References

Agency for Healthcare Research and Quality. (2012). *Defining the PCMH*. https://www.ahrq.gov/ncepcr/research/care-coordination/pcmh/define.html

Albee, G. W. (1998). Fifty years of clinical psychology: Selling our soul to the devil. *Applied & Preventive Psychology, 7*(3), 189–194. https://doi.org/10.1016/S0962-1849(05)80021-6

Anderson, J. A., & Doherty, W. J. (2005). Democratic community initiatives: The case of overscheduled kids. *Family Relations, 54*(5), 654–665. https://doi.org/10.1111/j.1741-3729.2005.00349.x

Aubel, J. (2022). Promoting community-driven change in family and community systems to support girls' holistic development in Senegal. In G. Palmer, T. Rogers, J. Viola, & M. Engel (Eds.), *Case studies in community psychology practice: A global lens* (pp. 64–86). Creative Commons.

Bailey, B. L., & Farber, D. E. (2004). (Eds.). *America in the seventies.* University Press of Kansas.

Baron, H., Blair, R. A., Choi, D. D., Gamboa, L., Gottlieb, J., Robinson, A. L., Rosenzweig, S. C., Turnbull, M. M., & West, E. A. (2021). *Can Americans depolarize? Assessing the effects of reciprocal group reflection on partisan polarization.* OSF Preprints. https://doi.org/10.31219/osf.io/3x7z8

Baron, N., Jensen, S., & de Jong, J. (2003). Refugees and internally displaced people. In B. L. Green, M. J. Friedman, J. de Jong, S. D. Solomon, T. M. Keane, J. A. Fairbank, B. Donelan, E. Frey-Wouters, & Y. Danieli (Eds.), *Trauma interventions in war and peace: Prevention, practice, and policy* (pp. 243–270). Springer. https://doi.org/10.1007/978-0-306-47968-7_11

Beckett, K. (1999). *Making crime pay: Law and order in contemporary American politics.* Oxford University Press.

Behnke, A. O., & Allen, W. D. (2007). Effectively serving low-income fathers of color. *Marriage & Family Review, 42*(2), 29–50. https://doi.org/10.1300/J002v42n02_03

Berge, J. M., Jin, S. W., Hanson, C., Doty, J., Jagaraj, K., Braaten, K., & Doherty, W. J. (2016). Play it forward! A community-based participatory research approach to childhood obesity prevention. *Families, Systems, & Health, 34*(1), 15–30. https://doi.org/10.1037/fsh0000116

Berge, J. M., Mendenhall, T. J., & Doherty, W. J. (2009). Using community-based participatory research (CBPR) to target health disparities in families. *Family Relations, 58*(4), 475–488. https://doi.org/10.1111/j.1741-3729.2009.00567.x

Bertoa, F. C., & Rama, J. (2021). Polarization: What do we know and what can we do about it? *Frontiers of Political Science, 3.* https://doi.org/10.3389/fpos.2021.687695

Bogenschneider, K. (in press). *Family policy matters: How policymaking affects families and what professionals can do* (4th ed.). Routledge.

Boyte, H. C. (2004). *Everyday politics: Reconnecting citizens and public life.* University of Pennsylvania Press. https://doi.org/10.9783/9780812204216

Boyte, H. C., & Kari, N. (1996). *Building America: The democratic promise of public work.* Temple University Press.

Boyte, H., Kari, N., Lewis, J., Skelton, N., & O'Donoghue, J. (2000). *Creating the commonwealth: Public politics and the philosophy of public work.* Kettering.

Boyte, H. C., Ström, M.-L., Tranvik, I., Moore, T. L., O'Connor, S., & Patterson, D. R. (2018). *Awakening democracy through public work: Pedagogies of empowerment.* Vanderbilt University Press. https://doi.org/10.2307/j.ctv167595x

Braver Angels. (2017). *Who we are: A message from Trump and Clinton supporters from southwest Ohio.*

Brint, S., & Levy, C. S. (1999). Professions and civic engagement: Trends in rhetoric and practice, 1875-1995. In T. Skocpol & M. P. Fiorina (Eds.), *Civic engagement in American democracy* (pp. 163–210). Brookings Institution.

Brookes, G., & Harvey, K. (2015). Peddling a semiotics of fear: A critical examination of scare tactics and commercial strategies in public health promotion. *Social Semiotics, 25*(1), 57–80. https://doi.org/10.1080/10350330.2014.988920

Brown, C. (2021). Critical clinical social work and the neoliberal constraints on social justice in mental health. *Research on Social Work Practice, 31*(6), 644–652. https://doi.org/10.1177/1049731520984531

Brown, S. L., Nobiling, B. D., Teufel, J., & Birch, D. A. (2011). Are kids too busy? Early adolescents' perceptions of discretionary activities, overscheduling, and stress. *The Journal of School Health, 81*(9), 574–580. https://doi.org/10.1111/j.1746-1561.2011.00629.x

Brush, B. L., Mentz, G., Jensen, M., Jacobs, B., Saylor, K. M., Rowe, Z., Israel, B. A., & Lachance, L. (2020). Success in long-standing community-based participatory research (CBPR) partnerships: A scoping literature review. *Health Education & Behavior, 47*(4), 556–568. https://doi.org/10.1177/1090198119882989

Bryant-Lukosius, D., Spichiger, E., Martin, J., Stoll, H., Kellerhals, S. D., Fliedner, M., Grossmann, F., Henry, M., Herrmann, L., Koller, A., Schwendimann, R., Ulrich, A., Weibel, L., Callens, B., & De Geest, S. (2016). Framework for evaluating the impact of advanced practice nursing roles. *Journal of Nursing Scholarship, 48*(2), 201–209. https://doi.org/10.1111/jnu.12199

Chasin, R., Herzig, M., Roth, S., Chasin, L., Becker, C., & Stains, R. R., Jr. (1996). From diatribe to dialogue on divisive public issues: Approaches drawn from family therapy. *Mediation Quarterly, 13*(4), 323–344. https://doi.org/10.1002/crq.3900130408

Clark, A. K., & Eisenstein, M. A. (2013). Interpersonal trust: An age-period-cohort analysis revisited. *Social Science Research, 42*(2), 361–375. https://doi.org/10.1016/j.ssresearch.2012.09.006

Clarke, G. M., Conti, S., Wolters, A. T., & Steventon, A. (2019). Evaluating the impact of healthcare interventions using routine data. *BMJ, 365*, l2239. https://doi.org/10.1136/bmj.l2239

Cohen, L. (2008). *A consumers' republic: The politics of mass consumption in post-war America.* Viking.

Comas-Díaz, L. (2020). Liberation psychotherapy. In L. Comas-Díaz & E. Torres-Rivera (Eds.), *Liberation psychology: Theory, method, practice, and social justice* (pp. 169–185). American Psychological Association. https://doi.org/10.1037/0000198-010

D'Alonzo, K. T. (2010). Getting started in CBPR: Lessons in building community partnerships for new researchers. *Nursing Inquiry, 17*(4), 282–288. https://doi.org/10.1111/j.1440-1800.2010.00510.x

Deivanayagam, T. A., Lasoye, S., Smith, J., & Selvarajah, S. (2021). Policing is a threat to public health and human rights. *BMJ Global Health, 6*(2), e004582. https://doi.org/10.1136/bmjgh-2020-004582

Doherty, W. J. (1995). *Soul searching: Why psychotherapy must promote moral responsibility.* Basic Books.

Doherty, W. J. (2000). *Take back your kids: Confident parenting in turbulent times.* Sorin Books.

Doherty, W. J. (2003, September/October). See how they run: When did childhood turn into a rat race? *Psychotherapy Networker*, pp. 38–46, 63.

Doherty, W. J. (2022). *The ethical lives of clients: Transcending self-interest in psychotherapy.* American Psychological Association. https://doi.org/10.1037/0000263-000

Doherty, W. J., & Beaton, J. M. (2000). Family therapists, community, and civic renewal. *Family Process, 39*(2), 149–161. https://doi.org/10.1111/j.1545-5300.2000.39201.x

Doherty, W. J., & Carlson, B. Z. (2002). *Putting family first.* Henry Holt.

Doherty, W. J., & Carroll, J. S. (2007). Families and therapists as citizens: The Families and Democracy Project. In E. Aldarondo (Ed.), *Advancing social justice through clinical practice* (pp. 225–244). Lawrence Erlbaum Associates.

Doherty, W. J., & Mendenhall, T. (2006). Citizen health care: A model for engaging patients, families, and communities as co-producers of health. *Families, Systems, and Health, 24*(3), 251–263. https://doi.org/10.1037/1091-7527.24.3.251

Doherty, W. J., Mendenhall, T., & Berge, J. (2014). *Citizen health care* [White paper]. National Science Foundation.

Doherty, W. J., Mendenhall, T. J., & Berge, J. M. (2010). The Families and Democracy and Citizen Health Care Project. *Journal of Marital and Family Therapy, 36*(4), 389–402. https://doi.org/10.1111/j.1752-0606.2009.00142.x

Dusheck, J. (2016, April). Smokers have harder time getting jobs, study says. *Stanford Medicine News Center.* https://med.stanford.edu/news/all-news/2016/04/smokers-have-harder-time-getting-jobs-study-finds.html

Dyson, M. E. (2020). *Long time coming: Reckoning with race in America.* St. Martin's Press.

Dzur, A. W. (2008). *Democratic professionalism: Citizen participation and the reconstruction of professional ethics, identity, and practice.* Pennsylvania State Press.

Dzur, A. W. (2017). *Rebuilding public institutions together: Professionals and citizens in a participatory democracy.* Cornell Selects.

Eaton, A. A., Grzanka, P. R., Schlehofer, M. M., & Silka, L. (2021). Public psychology: Introduction to the special issue. *American Psychologist, 76*(8), 1209–1216. https://doi.org/10.1037/amp0000933

Eichstaedt, J. C., Sherman, G. T., Giorgi, S., Roberts, S. O., Reynolds, M. E., Ungar, L. H., & Guntuku, S. C. (2021). The emotional and mental health impact of the murder of George Floyd on the US population. *Proceedings of the National Academy of Sciences of the United States of America, 118*(39), e2109139118. https://doi.org/10.1073/pnas.2109139118

Erkens, C. (2019). *The handbook for collaborative common assessments: Tools for design, delivery, and data analysis.* Solution Tree Press.

Finkel, E. J., Bail, C. A., Cikara, M., Ditto, P. H., Iyengar, S., Klar, S., Mason, L., McGrath, M. C., Nyhan, B., Rand, D. G., Skitka, L. J., Tucker, J. A., Van Bavel, J. J., Wang, C. S., & Druckman, J. N. (2020). Political sectarianism in America. *Science, 370*(6516), 533–536. https://doi.org/10.1126/science.abe1715

Fredricks, J. A., & Simpkins, S. D. (2012). Promoting positive youth development through organized after-school activities: Taking a closer look at participation of ethnic minority youth. *Child Development Perspectives, 6*(3), 280–287. https://doi.org/10.1111/j.1750-8606.2011.00206.x

Friedman, C., Wyatt, J., & Ash, J. (2021). *Evaluation methods in biomedical and health informatics* (3rd ed.). Springer.

Goodman, A., Morgan, R., Kuehilke, R., & Fleming, K. (2018). "We've been researched to death": Exploring the research experiences of urban Indigenous peoples in Vancouver, Canada. *International Indigenous Policy Journal, 9*(2), 1–23. https://doi.org/10.18584/iipj.2018.9.2.3

Graffigna, G. (Ed.). (2017). *Transformative healthcare practice through patient engagement.* IGI Global. https://doi.org/10.4018/978-1-5225-0663-8

Grembowski, D. (2015). *The practice of health program evaluation* (2nd ed.). Sage.

Guttman, N., & Salmon, C. T. (2004). Guilt, fear, stigma and knowledge gaps: Ethical issues in public health communication interventions. *Bioethics, 18*(6), 531–552. https://doi.org/10.1111/j.1467-8519.2004.00415.x

Haas, S. (2005). *Smoking at the HHH Job Corps in St. Paul, MN.* Unpublished data.

Hetherington, M., & Weiler, J. (2018). *Prius or pickup: How the answers to four simple questions explain America's great divide.* Houghton Mifflin Harcourt.

Hillman, J., & Ventura, M. (1993). *We've had a hundred years of psychotherapy—and the world's getting worse.* HarperOne.

The HistoryMakers. (2006, February 16). *Thelma Gibson's biography.* https://www.thehistorymakers.org/biography/thelma-gibson-41

Honore, C. (2009). *Under pressure: Rescuing our children from the culture of hyper-parenting.* HarperOne.

Imber-Black, E. (1988). *Families and larger systems: A family therapist's guide through the labyrinth.* Guilford Press.

Israel, B., Eng, E., Schulz, A., & Parker, E. (Eds.). (2005). *Methods in community-based participatory research for health.* Jossey-Bass.

Jarvis, T. (2016). *From human doing to human being: Getting back to basics and tuning into yourself again.* Tash Jarvis.

Klein, E. (2020). *Why we're polarized.* Simon & Schuster.

Krishnan, A., Tandon, R., & Nongkynrih, B. (2020). Relevance of community-based participatory research in community medicine training. *Indian Journal of Community Medicine, 45*(3), 256–260. https://doi.org/10.4103/ijcm.IJCM_343_19

Kuehn, B. M. (2014). Criminal justice becomes front line for mental health care. *JAMA, 311*(19), 1953–1954. https://doi.org/10.1001/jama.2014.4578

Kuhfeld, M., Elizabeth Gershoff, E., & Paschall, K. (2018). The development of racial/ethnic and socioeconomic achievement gaps during the school years. *Journal of Applied Developmental Psychology, 57*(July–August), 62–73. https://doi.org/10.1016/j.appdev.2018.07.001

Lee, C. C. (Ed.). (2013). *Multicultural issues in counseling: New approaches to diversity* (4th ed.). American Counseling Association.

Lee, C. C. (Ed.). (2018). *Counseling for social justice* (3rd ed.). American Counseling Association Foundation.

Legette, K. B., Rogers, L. O., & Warren, C. A. (2022). Humanizing student–teacher relationships for Black children: Implications for teachers' social-emotional training. *Urban Education, 57*(2), 278–288. https://doi.org/10.1177/0042085920933319

Mason, L. (2018). Ideologues without issues: The polarizing consequences of ideological identities. *Public Opinion Quarterly, 82*(S1), 866–887. https://doi.org/10.1093/poq/nfy005

McDaniel, S. H., Doherty, W. J., & Hepworth, J. (2014). *Medical family therapy and integrated care* (2nd ed.). American Psychological Association. https://doi.org/10.1037/14256-000

McIntyre, A. (2008). *Participatory action research.* Sage.

McLaughlin, A. M. (2002). Social work's legacy: Irreconcilable differences? *Clinical Social Work Journal, 30*(2), 187–198. https://doi.org/10.1023/A:1015297529215

Mendenhall, T. (2021, May/June). Community wisdom: Walking in balance with Indigenous cultures. *Psychotherapy Networker*, 28–33. https://www.psychotherapynetworker.org/article/community-wisdom

Mendenhall, T., Berge, J., & Doherty, W. (2014). Engaging communities as partners in research: Advancing integrated care through purposeful partnerships. In J. Hodgson, A. Lamson, T. Mendenhall, & D. R. Crane (Eds.), *Medical family therapy: Advanced applications* (pp. 259–282). Springer. https://doi.org/10.1007/978-3-319-03482-9_14

Mendenhall, T. J., Berge, J. M., Harper, P., GreenCrow, B., LittleWalker, N., WhiteEagle, S., & BrownOwl, S. (2010). The Family Education Diabetes Series (FEDS): Community-based participatory research with a midwestern American Indian community. *Nursing Inquiry*, *17*(4), 359–372. https://doi.org/10.1111/j.1440-1800.2010.00508.x

Mendenhall, T., & Doherty, W. (2003). Partners in Diabetes: A collaborative, democratic initiative in primary care. *Families, Systems & Health*, *21*(3), 329–335. https://doi.org/10.1037/1091-7527.21.3.329

Mendenhall, T., & Doherty, W. (2007a). The ANGELS (A Neighbor Giving Encouragement, Love and Support): A collaborative project for teens with diabetes. In D. Linville & K. Hertlein (Eds.), *The therapist's notebook for family healthcare* (pp. 91–101). Hayworth Press.

Mendenhall, T. J., & Doherty, W. J. (2007b). Partners in Diabetes: Action research in a primary care setting. *Action Research*, *5*(4), 378–406. https://doi.org/10.1177/1476750307083722

Mendenhall, T., Doherty, W., Baird, M., & Berge, J. (2008). Citizen Health Care: Engaging patients, families, and communities as coproducers of health. *Minnesota Physician*, *21*(12), 1–13.

Mendenhall, T., Doherty, W., Berge, J., Fauth, J., & Tremblay, G. (2013). Community-based participatory research: Advancing integrated behavioral health care through novel partnerships. In M. R. Talen & A. B. Valeras (Eds.), *Integrated behavioral health in primary care: Evaluating the evidence, identifying the essentials* (pp. 99–130). Springer. https://doi.org/10.1007/978-1-4614-6889-9_6

Mendenhall, T., Doherty, W., LittleWalker, E., & Berge, J. (2018). Medical family therapy in community engagement. In T. Mendenhall, A. Lamson, J. Hodgson, and M. Baird (Eds.), *Clinical methods in medical family therapy* (pp. 401–429). Springer.

Mendenhall, T. J., Gagner, N. E., & Hunt, Q. A. (2015). A call to engage youth in health research. *Families, Systems, & Health*, *33*(4), 410–412. https://doi.org/10.1037/fsh0000163

Mendenhall, T. J., Harper, P. G., Henn, L., Rudser, K. D., & Schoeller, B. P. (2014). Community-based participatory research to decrease smoking prevalence in a high-risk young adult population: An evaluation of the Students Against Nicotine and Tobacco Addiction (SANTA) project. *Families, Systems, & Health*, *32*(1), 78–88. https://doi.org/10.1037/fsh0000003

Mendenhall, T., Harper, P., Stephenson, H., & Haas, S. (2011). The SANTA Project (Students Against Nicotine and Tobacco Addiction): Using community-based participatory research to improve health in a high-risk young adult population. *Action Research, 9*(2), 199–213. https://doi.org/10.1177/1476750310388051

Mendenhall, T. J., Seal, K. L., GreenCrow, B. A., LittleWalker, K. N., & BrownOwl, S. A. (2012). The Family Education Diabetes Series: Improving health in an urban-dwelling American Indian community. *Qualitative Health Research, 22*(11), 1524–1534. https://doi.org/10.1177/1049732312457469

Mendenhall, T., Whipple, H., Harper, P., & Haas, S. (2008). Students Against Nicotine and Tobacco Addiction (SANTA): Developing novel interventions in smoking cessation through community-based participatory research. *Families, Systems, & Health, 26*(2), 225–231. https://doi.org/10.1037/1091-7527.26.2.225

Meyer, M. L., Louder, C. N., & Nicolas, G. (2021). Creating *with*, not *for* people: Theory of change and logic models for culturally responsive community-based intervention. *American Journal of Evaluation, 43*(3), 378–393. https://doi.org/10.1177/10982140211016059

Miami-Dade County. (2021). *Thrive305 Survey findings.* https://www.miamidade.gov/resources/pdf/thrive-305-preliminary-survey-findings.pdf

Michalek, A. K., Wong, S. L., Brown-Johnson, C. G., & Prochaska, J. J. (2020). Smoking and unemployment: A photo elicitation project. *Tobacco Use Insights, 13.* https://doi.org/10.1177/1179173X20921446

Miles, J. R., & Fassinger, R. E. (2021). Creating a public psychology through a scientist–practitioner–advocate training model. *American Psychologist, 76*(8), 1232–1247. https://doi.org/10.1037/amp0000855

Moore, G. F., Audrey, S., Barker, M., Bond, L., Bonell, C., Hardeman, W., Moore, L., O'Cathain, A., Tinati, T., Wight, D., & Baird, J. (2015). Process evaluation of complex interventions: Medical Research Council guidance. *BMJ, 350*, h1258. https://doi.org/10.1136/bmj.h1258

National Job Corps Association. (2023). *Job Corps works for at-risk youth.* https://njcaweb.org/job-corps-works/at-risk-youth

Neufeld, S. D., Chapman, J., Crier, N., Marsh, S., McLeod, J., & Deane, L. A. (2019). Research 101: A process for developing local guidelines for ethical research in heavily researched communities. *Harm Reduction Journal, 16*, 41. https://doi.org/10.1186/s12954-019-0315-5

Nieveen, N., & Folmer, E. (2013). Formative evaluation in educational design research. In T. Plomp & N. Nieveen (Eds.), *Educational design research* (pp. 154–170). Netherlands Institute for Curriculum Development.

Nutting, P. A., Crabtree, B. F., Miller, W. L., Stange, K. C., Stewart, E., & Jaén, C. (2011). Transforming physician practices to patient-centered medical homes: Lessons from the national demonstration project. *Health Affairs (Project Hope), 30*(3), 439–445. https://doi.org/10.1377/hlthaff.2010.0159

Onookome-Okome, T., Gorondensky, J., Rose, E., Sauer, J., Lum, K., & Moodie, E. M. (2022). Characterizing patterns in police stops by race in Minneapolis from 2016 to 2021. *Journal of Ethnicity in Criminal Justice, 20*(2), 142–164. https://doi.org/10.1080/15377938.2022.2086192

Pasick, R. (2018, June 25). *I am public psychologist: What does that mean?* https://robpasick.com/i-am-public-psychologist-what-does-that-mean

Phinney, J. (1992). The Multigroup Ethnic Identity Measure: A new scale for use with diverse groups. *Journal of Adolescent Research, 7*, 156–176.

Powell, R. (2006). *Evaluation research: An overview.* Johns Hopkins University Press.

Prochaska, J. J., Michalek, A. K., Brown-Johnson, C., Daza, E. J., Baiocchi, M., Anzai, N., Rogers, A., Grigg, M., & Chieng, A. (2016). Likelihood of unemployed smokers vs nonsmokers attaining reemployment in a one-year observational study. *JAMA Internal Medicine, 176*(5), 662–670. https://doi.org/10.1001/jamainternmed.2016.0772

Putnam, R. D. (2001). *Bowling alone: The collapse and revival of American community.* Simon & Schuster.

Putnam, R. D. (2020). *The upswing: How America came together a century ago and how we can do it again.* Simon & Schuster.

Redding, R. E. (2001). Sociopolitical diversity in psychology. The case for pluralism. *American Psychologist, 56*(3), 205–215. https://doi.org/10.1037/0003-066X.56.3.205

Reibling, N. (2016). The patient-centered medical home: How is it related to quality and equity among the general adult population? *Medical Care Research and Review, 73*(5), 606–623. https://doi.org/10.1177/1077558715622913

Ridley, M., Rao, G., Schilbach, F., & Patel, V. (2020). Poverty, depression, and anxiety: Causal evidence and mechanisms. *Science, 370*(6522). https://doi.org/10.1126/science.aay0214

Salabarría-Peña, Y., Apt, B. S., & Walsh, C. M. (2007). *Practical use of program evaluation among sexually transmitted disease (STD) programs.* Centers for Disease Control and Prevention. https://www.cdc.gov/std/program/pupestd.htm

Saul, J. (2000). Mapping trauma: A multi-systemic approach. In *Psychosocial notebook: Vol. 1. Psychosocial and trauma response in war-torn societies* (pp. 103–110). International Organization for Migration. https://publications.iom.int/system/files/pdf/ptr_kosovo_en.pdf

Saul, J. (2022). *Collective trauma, collective healing: Promoting community resilience in the aftermath of disaster.* Taylor & Francis.

Seal, K., Blum, M., Didericksen, K., Mendenhall, T., Gagner, N., GreenCrow, B., LittleWalker, K., BrownOwl, S., & Benton, K. (2016). The East Metro American Indian Diabetes Initiative: Engaging Indigenous men in reclaiming health and spirituality through community-based participatory research. *Journal of Health Education Research & Development, 4*(1), 152. https://doi.org/10.4172/2380-5439.1000152

Shaw, B., Kohli, A., & Igras, S. (2020). *Grandmother Project—Change through culture: Girls' holistic development program quantitative research report.* Institute for Reproductive Health, Georgetown University, with the United States Agency for International Development (USAID). https://www.irh.org/resource-library/ghd-quant-report

Simply Well Balanced. (2022, May 6). *10 simple tips for throwing a stress free birthday party.* https://simply-well-balanced.com/stress-free-simple-kids-birthday-party-ideas

Skenaz, L. (2021). *Free-range kids: How parents and teachers can let go and let grow.* Jossey-Bass.

Steele, C. M., Spencer, S. J., & Aronson, J. (2002). Contending with group image: The psychology of stereotype and social identity threat. *Advances in Experimental Social Psychology, 34*, 379–440. https://doi.org/10.1016/S0065-2601(02)80009-0

Stringer, E., & Aragon, A. (2021). *Action research* (5th ed.). Sage.

Sukarieh, M., & Tanhock, S. (2013). On the problem of over-researched communities: The case of the Shatila Palestinian refugee camp in Lebanon. *Sociology, 47*(3), 494–508. https://doi.org/10.1177/0038038512448567

Sullivan, W. M. (2004). *Work and integrity: The promise and crisis of professionalism in America* (2nd ed.). Jossey-Bass.

Taylor, E., Guy-Walls, P., Wilkerson, P., & Addae, R. (2019). The historical perspectives of stereotypes on African-American males. *Journal of Human Rights and Social Work, 4*(3), 213–225. https://doi.org/10.1007/s41134-019-00096-y

Tervalon, M., & Murray-Garcia, J. (1998). Cultural humility versus cultural competence: A critical distinction in defining physician training outcomes in multicultural education. *Journal of Health Care for the Poor and Underserved, 9*(2), 117–125. https://doi-org/10.1353/hpu.2010.0233

Woodland, M. H. (2008). Whatcha doin' after school? A review of the literature on the influence of after-school programs on young Black males. *Urban Education, 43*(5), 537–560. https://doi.org/10.1177/0042085907311808

Index

About the Authors

William J. Doherty, PhD, is a professor in the Department of Family Social Science at the University of Minnesota, where he directs the Citizen Professional Center and the Minnesota Couples on the Brink Project. In his career he has combined clinical innovations, including the specialties of medical family therapy and discernment counseling for couples on the brink of divorce, with a wide range of community engagement projects. In 2016 he cofounded Braver Angels, a national initiative to counteract polarization and restore the fraying social fabric of the nation. Among his awards is the Lifetime Achievement Award from the American Family Therapy Academy.

Tai J. Mendenhall, PhD, is a medical family therapist and professor in the Couple and Family Therapy Program at the University of Minnesota (UMN) in the Department of Family Social Science. He is an adjunct professor in the UMN's Department of Family Medicine and Community Health. Tai is also the director of the UMN's Medical Reserve Corps' Behavioral Health Response Strike Team and the associate director of the UMN's Citizen Professional Center. He actively works in the conduct of integrated and collaborative family health care, training, and outreach. His efforts in community-based participatory research and citizen health care initiatives center on a variety of public health issues.